THE ART OF
Tantra

THE ANCIENT SECRETS OF SEXUAL ENERGY AND SPIRITUAL GROWTH REVEALED

GUILLERMO FERRARA

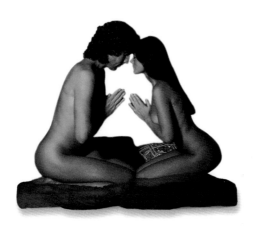

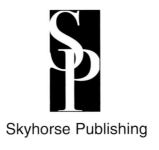

Skyhorse Publishing

Original title: EL ARTE DEL TANTRA
© Guillermo Ferrara
© Editorial Océano, S.L.
(Barcelona, Spain)

Skyhorse Publishing books may be purchased in bulk at special discounts for sales promotion, corporate gifts, fund-raising, or educational purposes. Special editions can also be created to specifications. For details, contact the Special Sales Department, Skyhorse Publishing, 307 West 36th Street, 11th Floor, New York, NY 10018 or info@skyhorsepublishing.com.

Skyhorse® and Skyhorse Publishing® are registered trademarks of Skyhorse Publishing, Inc.®, a Delaware corporation.

Visit our website at www.skyhorsepublishing.com.

10 9 8 7 6 5 4 3 2

Library of Congress Cataloging-in-Publication Data

Ferrara, Guillermo.
[Arte del tantra. English]
The art of tantra : the ancient secrets of sexual energy and spiritual
growth revealed / Guillermo Ferrara.
pages cm
ISBN 978-1-63220-491-2 (paperback) – ISBN 978-1-63220-746-3 (ebook) 1.
Sex instruction–Religous aspects–Tantrism. 2. Meditation–Tantric Buddhism.
3. Tantrism. I. Title.
HQ64.F4613 2015
294.5'514–dc23
2015015655

Cover design by Laura Klynstra
Cover photo credit: Thinkstock

Print ISBN: 978-1-63220-491-2
Ebook ISBN: 978-1-63220-746-3

Printed in China

*To my mother and father, and to the
long line of descendents in the family
tree, for completing that sacred sexual
act of which I am a product.*

AUTHOR'S NOTE

*Before beginning this book, I want to tell you the most important things I have learned in
my tantric experience:*

1. Minds are like parachutes: they only work when they're open.

*2. Morality, guilt, repression, and sexual taboos are unnatural impositions created by various religions and governments to control you; you don't belong to them. Don't judge,
just observe.*

*3. You are free, you were born to feel pleasure, to evolve and be creative, to fill your
soul with joy through meditative sex, through laughter and dance, filling every day
of your life.*

CONTENTS

INTRODUCTION

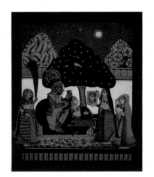

W e often forget about our deepest self, buried under schedules, worries, work, unresolved emotional problems, fears, and a whole array of distractions that distance us from our hearts.

Men and women can now free themselves from all these internal conflicts with a single shift in their perspective on life. Sometimes you only see the negative side of existence and forget that everything has a sense of growth.

Tantra is a complete science of human life, in all its dimensions. Some have branded it as only a path to sex without seeing that it goes so much farther. It's as if we only see a tree, missing the whole forest.

This book will attempt to show the whole panorama that Tantra encompasses, being the result of a personal attempt to live honestly, practicing what I preach.

Within the existence of a person there is more than sex; there are also emotions, thoughts, ideas, plans, longings of the soul, and physical and spiritual growth. It just so happens that sex is one of the first rungs on the ladder in the evolution of the conscience, and if we want to climb a staircase, but don't take the first step, it will be difficult to get to the top. Yes, Tantra deals with sex, but in a simultaneously scientific and romantic way. It also deals with love, but with intelligence, and with material goods, but in enjoying them without becoming devoted to them or valuing them too much.

Many spiritual traditions have "left out" the subject of sex, while others have openly repressed and condemned it.

Think about it . . .

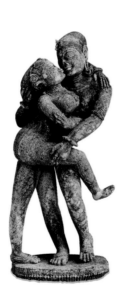

Haven't we all come into the world through a sexual act? Wasn't it necessary for two bodies to come together, in soul and energy, to produce a miraculous birth? Why stigmatize something so sacred as sinful? Is it that humanity has not understood that sex, more than generating a new life, is also a spiritual transformation?

Tantra knows that all of life is energy, and that it is all one energy that has different aspects. Sex is a very important one and, used wisely, can drive the purification and illumination of the spirit. But it can also take another road: perverse and mental, or repressed, like in some societies.

Tantra takes sex to be pleasure and a connection between two beings seeking to become one, the opening of a sacred door in the conscience leading to deep levels of understanding of natural forces. The sexual act is, ultimately, the microcosmic representation of the universal law of attraction—of the creation that unites the two poles.

Life is day and night, hot and cold, dry and wet, man and woman . . . In life, balance is a supreme law and Tantra is a path to balance: sex united with meditation, financial well-being compatible with spiritual exploration, happiness and fun together with moments of silence . . .

Tantra is practice, it is learning through direct experience. You raise your energy and soul, you observe with clarity and understand, you connect with life and you are happy. This path can be a lifesaver for the modern man, who walks aimlessly through life, or even for the wise one who realizes that "there's something more" to life than eating, sleeping, and lovemaking.

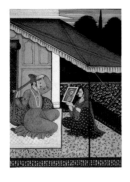

Tantra awakens an artistic capacity in the physical body; the common man travels the path to Buddha by bringing all his hidden potential to the surface. He does this by uncovering the heart, freeing it, giving it wings to live freely and consciously.

Without being a religion, it is a tapestry that includes all the facets of life without discarding a single one. You enjoy your belongings, discover the sanctity of sex, delight in food; you love and are loved, you become creative, you follow your intuition, and live from your center. Isn't that a perfect life? Can it be that we all hold the keys to happiness and are putting them in the wrong locks?

Tantra is a path of subtraction, not summation or division: remove what is unnecessary, just as the artist does from the stone, and allow the sculpture to emerge.

With Tantra, you don't arrive to any one place because it is not a race: it's an adventure and acceptance, it's the discovery of magical and powerful consciousness, it's the dance that every being dances, it's the page in which the poet captures their work, it's the recovery of joy and love in all its dimensions. It is like knocking on the door of your own house without knowing how many rooms are inside: the surprise of opening every room and discovering the light inside, seeing the divinity of every space, and feeling that you are a mirror that reflects life inside of you.

GUILLERMO FERRARA, Barcelona, September 2001

9

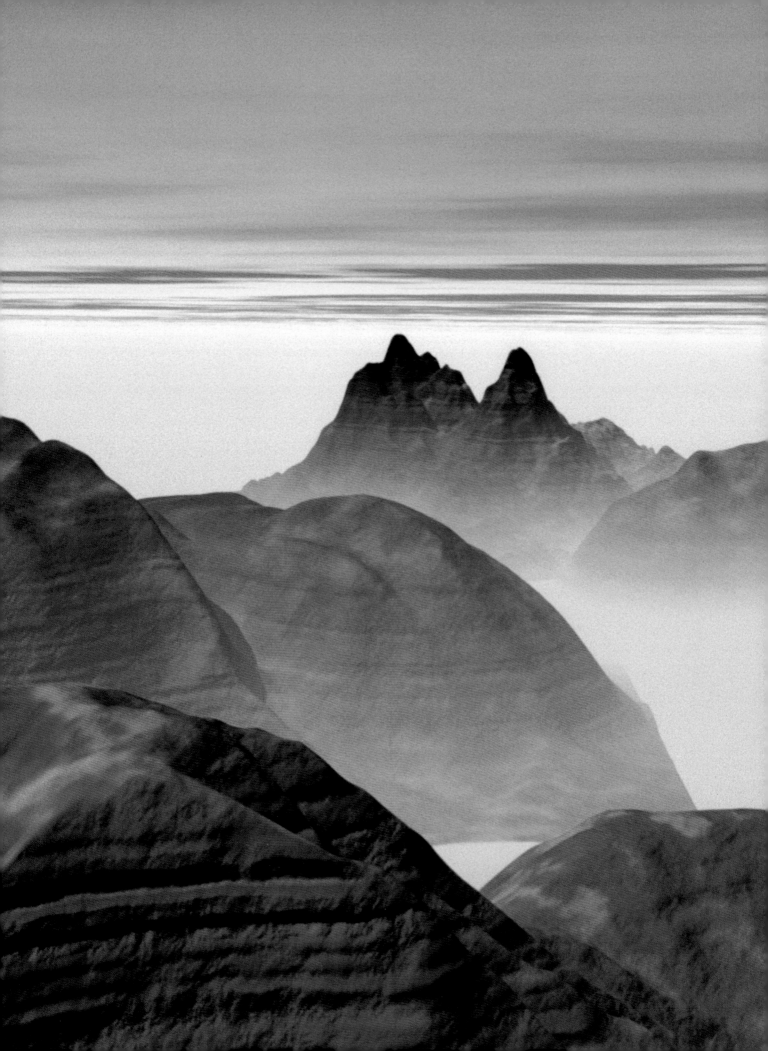

THE PSYCHOLOGY
OF TANTRA

*"Tantra is the beginning of a new human being,
scientific and spiritual, loving and meditative,
profound and sexual, that creates, with his energy,
a way of life approaching Heaven on Earth."*
OSHO

AWAKENING *Your* POTENTIAL

Many spiritual paths seek to liberate the soul. Tantra does this through ritual sex, which awakens the psychosexual energy that leads to enlightenment.

Tantra is a tool of human transformation, a path that originates in the body and leads to liberation. Various aspects of the body require attention to maintain health and increase energy flow in order to vibrate in harmony with the universe, which is itself a large body.

For Tantra, the physical body is the starting point in the spiritual search, the roots that allow you to reach the wings, the temple in which the individual lives the game of life (lilah).

While many systems of spirituality deny the body, desire, and sex (they consider it taboo, either from fear or because when you control sexual energy you rule all the energies of nature), Tantra accepts the body as sacred, desire as a bridge to transcendence, and sex as a source of pleasure, meditation, and spiritual ecstasy. This is a more intelligent way.

It is a school of thought that seeks complete liberty and the fulfillment of the individual on every plane. Its origin is matriarchal, not dogmatic or repressive, and its not subjected to

beliefs but rather based in the potential to learn through experience. There is an emphasis in the feminine power of life and therefore does not mutilate or condemn women as patriarchal systems do.

It is a spiritual and mystic science, but it is not a religion because it affirms that we are not isolated, that everything is connected. Therefore, it is unnecessary to regulate man, but

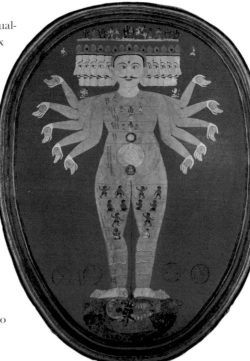

The universe as a cosmic man.

rather make him conscious that God is in everything, *is* everything.

Tantra immerses itself in life in harmony with the laws of nature, without being bound to any holy book (although there are essential tantric texts), in order to feel the experiences that lead to spiritual growth. It allows one to enter, body and soul, into life without being fragmented or thinking in dualities. It doesn't believe in good or evil, but rather in what is just and natural.

It attempts to encourage the individual to free his or herself from any and all psychic or emotional bondage and repression, and to be his or herself from his or her interior being (atma) rather than the false personality or ego (ahamkara).

Etymologically, "Tantra" means "woven for the expansion of consciousness," and as such includes multiple techniques in art, science, mysticism, yoga, dance, breathing, massages, spirituality, postures, and the wondrous focus on life. Its psychology is based in acting, feeling, and thinking from the soul (atma), on the same frequency as the divine or supreme soul (atman). There are two ways of

12

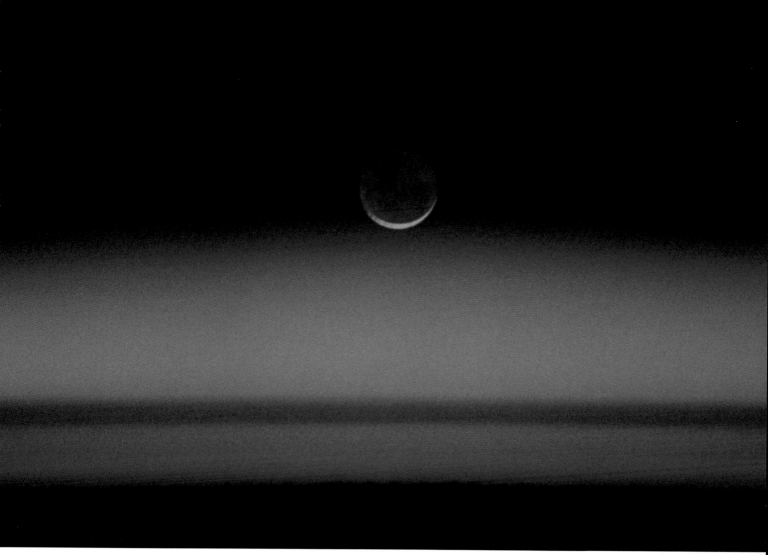

living: positive, connected with life, the universe, and nature (and therefore with love and the luminous vision of life), or the contrary, solitary, disconnected from existence, and fighting instead of learning. Youcan only live connected or disconnected. If you are connected, you will have the sensation that everything happens through an invisible hand that supports you in every moment and helps you grow. If not, you will feel isolated.

Tantra nowadays is a pragmatic path and easily accessible to the modern man with spiritual anxiety, because it does not involve an organized religion but rather a free and responsible path that allows for inner growth and enjoyment without guilt, remorse, or attachment.

THE ORIGIN OF TANTRA

Tantra (meaning "loom," "cloth," "treaty," or "system") is a spiritual way whose history began very long ago. Although its teachings were passed on through oral tradition, it also draws from some written texts, the oldest of which dates back to the 6th century BC.

The Tantras, such as are the sacred texts, are presumed to have been revealed by Shiva as writings specifically for the Kali Yuga (4th or current age of the world) and they offer private conversations between the god Shiva and his wife, the goddess Shakti. First, we hear the voice of Shiva as disciple, and then Shakti, together communicating to each other the secret essence. A central concept of Tantra is the adoration of the femi-

nine; Shakti as a divine manifestation of woman, also known as Davi, Durga, Kali, Parvati, Uma, Sati, Padma, Candi, Tripura Sundari, etc.

Tantra was developed mainly in India and from there spread to China and Tibet. There are various branches of Tantra: the branch on the right is Buddhist, characterized by an imaginary sexual relationship stressed through meditation; the left branch is Hindu, where the sex act is practiced along side other energy practices. This book focuses on neotantra, which leaves behind some of the rituals unfamiliar to the Western world and substitutes them with other practices from around the world while still allowing one to reach a state of expanded consciousness.

This book's approach is open to sexual relationships, so it can be considered more a part of the left branch; one that includes the making of mandalas, symbols, the use of consciousness and creative energy, breathing, movement of energy, and sexual practice directed toward sacred spaces of consciousness, in pursuit of unity between man and woman, Shiva and Shakti, the god and the goddess.

The *Vigyan Bhairava Tantra*, which means "technique to transcend consciousness," is a treatise that is over five thousand years old and describes 112 methods of meditation. It is a text in which Shiva gives tantric instructions to his consort, Devi, and we can see the principle female (Shakti) assume different roles, from that of lover, Great Mother, or Kali (she who destroys in order to rebuild).

The *Kularnava Tantra*, one of the main texts, reclaims the use of "the five M's," named for their initials in Sanskrit, which are the five elements used in sexual rituals, or maithuna: wine (madya) represents fire; meat (mamsa), air; fish (matsya), water; fruits and bread (mudra), earth; and the sex act (maithuna), space. In this way, the couple consumes foods while remaining conscious of this symbolism, to prepare for transcendence and the drawing in of reality.

The relation between Tantra and sex, made popular mainly through the diffusion of Oriental erotic art (mainly that of ancient India), attracted the interest of many in the West. This is primarily because in our civilization (which now covers most of the planet) sex has come to play a central role in our lives. One only has to look at commercial advertising to see that sex is used to sell products. But Tantra is not just sex: it teaches a total way of being for the self-actualization of the individual, as much through sexuality as through other spiritual means.

The sacred texts of Tantra are presumed to be told by Shiva and describe private conversations with his wife, Shakti.

WHAT IS THE AIM

"You are already perfect, you don't want to fight to be someone," said Osho, spiritual master of Tantra. There is no need to create inner conflict but rather flush out the darkness that hides the diamond and express ourselves. Tantra produces internal transformations that convert back into energy. It takes one from depression to celebration, from rigid to flexible, from critical and uncreative to blind conscious impulse. Through daily practice, you are always changing, evolving, because perfection does not have limits, nor is it static. Automobiles in the 1970s where perfect "for that time," the best of the time period, but those of today are far superior. Perfections are part of the "here and now."

Tantra aims for the complete development of the consciousness, free in every plane, and for this it does not reject the world or consider it an illusion, but rather something very real. Take the Earth as another school of life and she will teach you to enjoy every function of your energy. Tantra does not condemn sex, nor food, nor recreation, but rather, on the contrary, uses these things to climb higher.

14

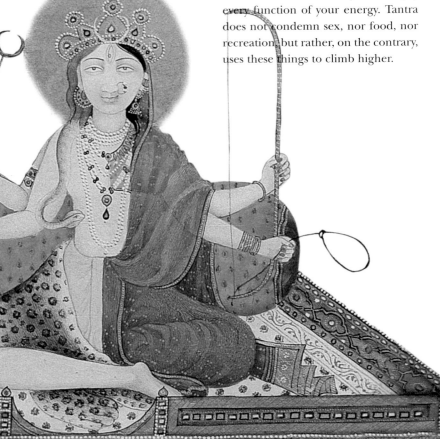

The unity of man and woman, Shiva and Shakti, is the central aim of Tantra.

The formula is a combination of consciousness and energy, sex and meditation, love and intelligence, creativity and sensuality, perception and celebration.

THE PRINCIPLE UNITY: SHIVA AND SHAKTI

Tantra is a holistic current (from "holos," "total," or "complete") that allows the individual to cross the bridge to sacred consciousness and enlightenment, supported by the mundane.

There is no division between the material and the spiritual because according to Tantra, all division is an illusion; we are all eternally united with the universe, the One, the Tao, the Absolute. Such is implied by the name we call it.

From the original unity, the field of energy transforms into two polarities, or duality: Shiva, the masculine, and Shakti, the feminine. Between both complementary opposites there is light. On a small scale, this phenomenon is observable in many ways: for example, in a plug, which has male and female components, the connection generates light through a cable, which would be life.

This principal of feminine-masculine is always in balance: woman and man, Moon and Sun, cold and heat, wet and dry, winter and summer, etc.

How to grasp the state of "consciousness of unity" if we apparently feel separated? First of all, it is important to be one with our inner man or woman. If we were to split the human body in two, we would find two hemispheres of the brain (one feminine and one masculine), two lungs, two eyes, two arms, two ovaries, two testicles, two kidneys, and two legs. These two parts function in harmony with each other and the cosmos; a balance of energetic function mirroring the principal unity, which can easily be reached by daily tantric practice, no miracle pills required.

TANTRIC DEITIES

Tantra relies on a trinity to explain the genesis of the cosmos: Brahma, Shiva, and Vishnu.

Brahma is the source of creations, *linked with the birth of all things and whose spouse is Saraswati, patroness of art.*

Shiva is considered the source of transcendence *and is linked with death. His spouse is Kali (who initiates the transcendent and the sexual) in her aspect of destruction.*

Vishnu, linked with conservation and the beginning of life, *has for his partner Lakshmi, incarnation of conservation and prosperity. A westerner should consider these names as familiar as principles such as birth, life, and death. The Mundaka Upanishad says: "Brahma, the Creator, wished that it were so and with his will created the beginning of the universe. From this came the first energy and from this, the mind. Then the subtle elements emerged and from these, the different worlds. With the acts performed by the beings of these worlds, the chain of cause and effect was established." He is the principle whom we would call the "Cosmic Father," as Brahma is directly related to continuous creation. The Saraswati Stotra says of his spouse, Saraswati: "Saraswati, the spouse of Brahma, has a corporeal glow more powerful than the light of ten million moons. Her robes are purified by the celestial fire. She is the Mother of the Vedas, the incarnation of nature and the patroness of art and science. She always smiles and is extremely beautiful, with a body decorated with jewels and pearls." She is the principle whom we call the "Cosmic Mother." In another sacred text we find the following: "Brahma began the process of creation, dividing himself into a man and a woman who made love. Brahma and Saraswati conceived together the race of mortals."*

Represented within the physical body, Brahma is food, Vishnu is drink,

and Shiva is breath. Together with their Shaktis, each one represents one of the senses. Lakshmi is touch; Brahma, sight; Kali, smell; Shiva, the mind; Saraswati, hearing; and Vishnu, taste. Finally, with respect to the subtle body where the nadis, or meridians, are: Brahma represents the right solar channel, or pingala; Vishnu, the left channel, or ida; and Shiva, the central channel, or sushumna. The pubis of the woman represents an inverted triangle—the yoni—with three points that are Lakshmi, Saraswati, and Kali. Similarly, in the man there is a triangle pointing upward; each point represents Shiva (the upper one), and Brahma and Vishnu (the base). The unity of material and the spirit produces a magic six-pointed star.

We see the characteristics of the goddesses in the contemporary woman:

KALI
With bright and powerful eyes, long unruly hair, and a sensual, erotic body, she is ready for sex at any moment. She represents the hidden and powerful side of Shakti (the spouse of Shiva) and is related to: the past, the present, and the future; the four cardinal points; primal nature and nudity; internal mysteries; destruction; ardent sexuality; and the new moon. She is the kundalini in its active state, wild and passionate love.

LAKSHMI
She is the stereotype of the sweet and gentle woman. Extremely sensual, she is the full moon and beauty in all her expressions.

SARASWATI
The artistic woman, master of the sixty-four tantric arts, she is beautiful, a lover of nature, smiling, and kind. She is wise and delicate.

Supreme deity, Shiva and Shakti is half man and half woman.

TANTRIC TRANSFORMATION

When you enter into the tantric consciousness, your view of the world changes; what was previously dark and shadowy, taboo, or fear, becomes light and manifests itself by transforming your heart and your perception. You stop being careless, cold, or distant; an inner fire (archetype of spiritual power) burns in you, alights the heart. The practice of Tantra makes you love the whole spectrum of life. You leave behind doubts, fears, and conflicts and you give in to adventure, uncertainty, confidence, and change. It is a giving in to the magical mystery of the universe.

> When you enter into the tantric consciousness, your view of the world changes; what was previously dark and shadowy, taboo, or fear, becomes light and transforms your heart and your perception.

The tantric transformation is so strong that your whole world changes. No one can dominate you, you cease to be a submissive person, and gain your own voice.

You begin to develop an inner power that heightens your intelligence and your love, and that expands your consciousness in order to understand the natural forms of life.

You cease to be bound; you achieve liberation, the happy manifestation of your creativity, the life impulse that leads in all directions. You laugh, you dance, you celebrate, and you enjoy life, this evolutionary step you get to live. And the most important part is that with Tantra, spiritual enlightenment can occur at any moment!

STEPS TO SPIRITUAL EVOLUTION

Tantric spirituality is not a rigid system because one does not follow a spiritual path guided by dogmas or commandments but rather by conscience and liberty. The search occurs day by day, depending on where you are in life.

Spiritual growth means harmonizing with life in the present, so we can see every experience as potential learning experiences to help us evolve. You only need to be attentive to these moments of growth.

Here you have some points that may guide you on your "ladder" to enlightenment. They are some of the symptoms that an individual may feel, from the lowest to the highest.

1. Depression, fear, unhappiness
Some people need to experience the worst of misfortune or suffering in order to awaken the soul. To feel depression or fear means living in a distressed state. It is a point of departure to seek another path.

2. Desire to change
When you realize that the path you're on is not leading to happiness or evolution, the desire to change takes over. Many people who meditate or who work on their inner growth want to encourage their loved ones to start, but if the desire to change is not there, if it does not come from the individual, they cannot receive these new energies.

3. Begin meditation and energetic practice
With the desire to change, you look for a strategy for transformation: a particular sadhana or energetic practice. There are many methods that can help you. Tantra is the science of energy and the art of living. At this point, the individual needs will power and discipline to change their condition.

Meditation, the asanas of yoga, dances, and special breaths allow your energy to begin to vibrate on new levels. It is important to know that everything that you emit, such as thoughts and emotions, is what you will receive. This step requires dynamic meditation in order to change your focus and bioenergetic polarity.

4. Catharsis: cleaning and cleansing
The effect of sadhana allows for the existence of an inner conflict. The old things (habits, beliefs, rigid thoughts, and self pitying emotions) will be pushed aside by new things. Catharsis

ELIGHTENMENT

Many spiritual paths seek, through different roads, Moksha, Nirvana, or Samadhi: the liberation of the personal soul and its fusion with the universal soul. The objective of tantric practice is also this enlightenment of consciousness, and it bases this on special techniques that achieve this awakening through the physical senses. Sexual activity is considered sadhana, a spiritual practice that offers the opportunity of enlightenment. It uses ritual sex, maithuna, to awaken the psychosexual energy, or kundalini, in the sacro-sexual region and make it rise along the astral column (sushumna) to the top of the head (to the crown chakra or sahasrara), provoking enlightenment. Obviously, like in all of nature, the changes are slight and take some time. Only catastrophes are sudden and thus destructive. Step by step, purifying the body, making it flexible and strong, nourishing it with energy (prana) through breathing exercises (pranayamas), physical poses (asanas) and dances, we will clean the nadis (the energy channels of the body), purifying emotions and thoughts, intensifying the sadhana (group or individual training) and working our way toward enlightenment.

is a war between the old, which resists, and the new, which wants to enter. Here the person may experience catharsis through a purifying cry, laughter, a state of openness, or euphoria. When this happens, one needs restraint and encouragement in order to see that the darkest, most threatening clouds can produce the purest, clearest rain.

5. Take consciousness. The observer is born.

This is a state in which the person feels as if they are on the landing of a spiral staircase. They take consciousness of all that they have been living and the "spool" begins to unravel. The taking of consciousness awakens the inner observer and allows one to see their own life like a movie. We grow wiser by seeing the errors of the past. This point is a breath after the catharsis.

6. Liberation of energy

Now most likely a liberation of energy will occur, and with it, new emotions, sensations, and flexible thoughts, both enthusiastic and creative.

7. Harmony

Here the seeker feels that their being is experiencing a state of harmony and balance. Harmony emerges because the energy becomes creative and flows through its natural channels. The mental and emotional aspects begin to harmonize. The inner processes and energy fill the body with health and vitality.

8. Deepening of meditation

After achieving harmony some people let it be and abandon their practice. However, harmony is a stage, not the goal, and one can quickly return to poor health. If you continue exercising, you can continue climbing, growing, and reaching new interior levels.

9. Inner peace

The result of continued practice is that the heart might find inner peace, even though this isn't a static state. Inner peace is more like breath: mobile, active, and always present—an oasis for the soul.

10. Expansion of the consciousness. Celebration and wisdom.

How distant all that suffering and depression seems now! This is the result of discipline and the elevation of energy. Now, the intuitive wisdom (prajna) vibrates in celebration, delight, and marvels in all that you experience daily. Your focus has changed radically because the inner eye has awoken and contemplates the light. Your inner state is now of the opposite polarity. We are now on a direct road toward ecstasy, toward the happiness hidden inside everyone, toward unity with All.

It is a state of illuminated consciousness where one is bathed in love and clarity. Here, the heart is the guide and all of nature is a sacred temple.

The spiritual evolution is a solitary, conscious, and happy path where you can enjoy, feel pleasure, and create in harmony with existence and all of the luminous beings. It is an adventure of the soul in search of a home where it belongs.

17

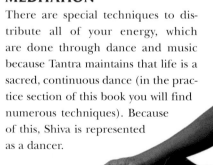

MUSIC, DANCE, AND MEDITATION

There are special techniques to distribute all of your energy, which are done through dance and music because Tantra maintains that life is a sacred, continuous dance (in the practice section of this book you will find numerous techniques). Because of this, Shiva is represented as a dancer.

Tantra affirms that absolutely everything is energy (from stone to vapor) in different phases. For example, if a person were depressed or unhappy, we would say that they have lower energy because it is stagnated in the first chakras. It needs to flow, and the dances, music, and cleansing or circular breaths will allow the energy to rise, and with it, their emotional and mental state. The techniques invoke a change that leads to balance. Through these techniques, the senses, which are windows to the soul and give pleasure, are awoken. In this way, you learn through pleasure and consciousness, rather than through suffering, through a road of happy Buddhas rather than serious saints.

With tantric dances, you enter into a state of deep meditation, leaving behind stress, repression and all of the false, unnatural beliefs imposed by the oppressive systems of humanity. Tantra makes your cells dance, makes your heart brim with enthusiasm and swell with desire to live. With dance, you feel free and stimulate the energy kundalini. You accept and love yourself.

THE TANTRIC CIRCLE OF ENERGY

Sex is taken as meditation.

The first sutra of Shiva with Devi says: "Upon entering in the sexual union, keep the attention fixed on the initial flame, without reaching the final embers."

There is no need to be in a hurry or rush to consummate desire and the sex act. The beginning of the union holds the spark and the fire, and the tantric maintains it so that it does not turn to coals and burn out. This is obtained through rhythm, creating a circle without beginning or end. In this way, you and your lover will feel as if you become a single wave of energy.

There is no need to think in the future or the past, because each time the flame emerges, the present is the only parameter with which to seek balance. This allows both to enjoy each other's bodies, the contact between the souls' energies, mixing one with the other in a circle.

If the sexual act is not hurried, it becomes spiritual; energy travels from the genital area to the entire body, avoiding any rush to ejaculate or reach orgasm.

There is no loss of energy but rather revitalization and togetherness. By accepting desire, the body and being cross the line from personal to transpersonal. The tantric circle dissolves the ego into a sea of consciousness.

The lovers generate light and energy like a dynamo. The energetic poles meet and connect the man's electricity with the woman's magnetism.

THE COSMIC TREMOR

The second sutra says: "When, in an embrace, you feel your senses shake like leaves, enter this tremor."

SEX

Tantrics have investigated and tested sexual energy for thousands of years through the ritual called maithuna. Contrary to the repressive Western teachings, Tantra claims that woman and man feel in harmony through this function of energy. It does not condemn sex, but encourages it! However, it is not debauchery, as it is considered an art, a science, and an access to the deepest levels of consciousness.

After all, who doesn't enjoy sexual pleasure? So, why repress it? Why let it be dominated or withheld? Here, sex deals with the sharing of energy without interference from the mind (with its false morals, its terms and conditions, and its erroneous beliefs), so that the kundalini (which is sacred and carries life) flows without guilt or thought of sin.

Tantra considers it very important that the man does not ejaculate because the energy that is released in ejaculation can be instead used to transform into **"vital oil."** This is called **ojas shakti**, which provides spiritual power so that the energy does not sink back into the earth but rather rises through the astral column and activates the seven chakras of consciousness. Through this activation the energy rises along with the perception of inner light like a door that opens to infinity.

Sexual energy is a source of pleasure, life, transformation, and of course, it is connected to consciousness and meditation. It is, no more or less, an artistic act in which each one is both artist and masterpiece. Tantra does not use sex for genital relief but rather an exchange of feminine energies (Shakti) with masculine ones (Shiva) in order to feel as one.

Tantra maintains that in the beginning we were androgynous, that is to say, one being that was half woman and half man. Sex (from sectus: "divide," "cut," "separate") was what provoked the game and the reunion to return to being one. Sex allows you to reunite with your other half in a state of being conscious of the unity of all. It is a representation on a small scale of higher laws.

Through the stimulation of sexual energy comes the manifestation of kundalini, which translates into creative acts, intuitions, better inspiration and impulse, more vitality, and capacity to know your inner processes, and is as such an inner power never before felt. The sacred energy, or kundalini, the manifestation of the feminine polarity of life, encircles you lovingly, making you more and more perceptive and conscious.

Three things may occur with sex: generation (the birth of a new being), degeneration (when energy takes an unnatural course), and regeneration (which is what Tantra proposes and which leads to a new birth, called dwij—he who was reborn, Buddha). This new birth was what Jesus said to the master Nicodemus. To be born with a new day-to-day focus, with a new understanding of the mysteries of life, the development of the talent that life has gifted you to execute, in love, in meditation, creating art like the universe . . . This internal birth means tuning in to the inner wisdom and the motor of this new birth is sexual energy. Don't forget that the whole world was born physically from a sex act, and that now you can be born spiritually, illuminating your destiny.

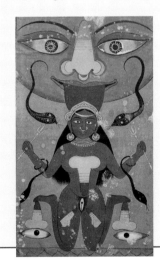

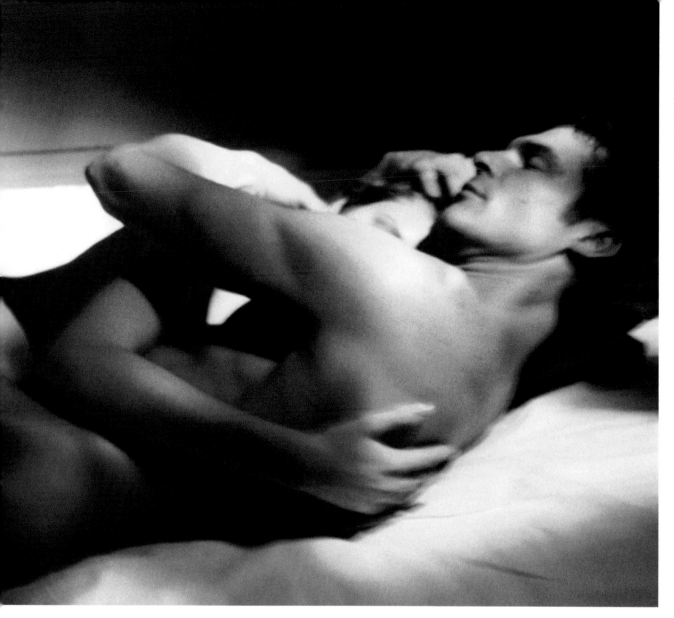

19

The tremor is a product of energy in motion; it makes the cells vibrate and opens the hidden emotional defenses through direct contact with the deepest essence of oneself: the spiritual heart.

The movement, the tremor, and the vibration of sex are used to light the serpentine fire that nourishes consciousness, the cells, and the body.

Sex is not mental but rather a real experience of bioenergies merging. With the tremor, energy runs along internal pathways, the circle is formed, and you can feel yourself as part of the universe, a universal cell of consciousness.

In the communion of a deep embrace, the senses are stimulated

A meditative attitude makes sex an experience that transcends carnal pleasure and eliminates fears and taboos.

and open like windows to the soul. You can remain in this state for hours. Existence is found in the present moment that you are living. The deep reality of unity is born in every individual and made whole in his or her self by sharing with a partner. You must move in sex with complete consciousness and alertness to what you are experiencing. The body is freed,

the mind silenced, the soul takes flight toward ecstasy.

For Tantra, making love is like a dance, an unfolding of energies that go from one body to the other as if entering a holy temple. A meditative attitude makes sex an experience that rises from carnal pleasure and stimulation of the senses, to feeling ones energy and the opening of the conscience while eliminating fears and taboos.

Shiva and Shakti, the man and the woman, recreate on a small scale the act of creation, where the forces of nature are recognized as complementary opposites: lovers as poles of the same field.

CONSCIOUSNESS AND ENERGY

Obviously, all important movement needs a center, a leader, an organizer. The enormous quantity of energy that is mobilized is governed by the consciousness. These two principles coexist in harmony in the universe. And for Tantra, it is vital to understand that the man is consciousness and the woman is energy. Consciousness and energy form the tantric base, the pillars that support its strategies.

Consciousness is the power of being awake. How many times have you crossed the street without realizing? How often are you thinking of one thing and doing another?

The great problem with people is that there is no deep consciousness, and almost all of the problems and woes are a result of this. For example, if a poor family has seven or ten children, it's very difficult for them to get ahead. If a driver drinks alcohol, it's very likely he will suffer an accident. When there is no consciousness, energy is low and problems arise. There's no point in having lots of energy if you are not conscious of it, since it will have no direction and will come out negatively.

All of the work of the spiritual search can be summed up as the need to expand the consciousness.

Imagine, for a moment, an example that will give you an idea of the objective: suppose that your consciousness is a circle with a diameter of 1

Tantra is not a philosophic path but rather an existential movement, consisting of growth through experience.

meter, and the cosmic consciousness has a diameter of 1,000 meters. If your consciousness begins to expand to 300, 500, up to 1,000 meters through meditation, then your own consciousness and that of the universe will have the same frequency and they will be one and the same.

There are specific exercises to increase energy and raise it through the chakras in order to expand the levels of consciousness.

GROWTH THROUGH DIRECT EXPERIENCE

Tantra is not a philosophic path but rather an existential movement, consisting of something as simple as growth through experience, to live by enjoying existence to the fullest.

The whole world has the same essence—the soul, the divinity that is within all of us—although not all of us have the same existence. Personality, experiences, talents, inclinations, abilities, intelligence, capacity to love and act . . . all of this makes up your individual existence and is different from other individuals.

To be existential means to eliminate the beliefs and replace them with direct experience. It's not talking about the benefits of water, but drinking it. Not reading magazines about exotic places but visiting them.

It has nothing to do with a fear of adventure but rather embracing adventure with the senses alert, an open heart, and wondering eyes. It has nothing to do with tradition either, doing the same thing generation upon generation, but rather to contribute your own particular genius, to collaborate with the universal existence and make it richer. It is an attitude toward life, an individual choice and free for each and every one of us.

Tantra is like the bed of a river; its course is always changing. All of the beliefs are dead if you don't try them for yourself. Life is constant change and existence is motion.

To synchronize the consciousness with this vibration is a job that Tantra wants you to do day by day, breath by breath. In fact, enlightenment is to be conscious of All in every moment: to be one with existence, without ego or division.

The divine essence, God, shares with you a seed of his existence; he gifts you your existence so you can enjoy it, so you can learn, and so you can play . . . make the most of it.

SEXUALITY AND STRESS

Tantra uses the sex act (maithuna) to communicate a message, to exchange the energy of love, to activate the chakras, and to raise the energy of the kundalini. It does not use sex to release tension. This can be released through physical activity such as dynamic meditation, going for a jog, or dancing. Tantric sex is something that goes much further.

When the body is relaxed, vibrant, healthy, alert, and ready to share energy, this is a useful state. Tantric techniques of breathing, the art of touch, of feeling, of caressing, of deepening into one another, all contribute to transport you to a unique,

eternal moment. It is eternal because it transcends time; your consciousness forgets about the clock and you fuse together for hours. When sex is used to relieve tension, there is relief, relaxation, and emptiness. But when it is used to share the heart and soul, you are filled with light, the body filled with peace and power, and the soul dances in delight.

A transformation occurs, a change in the way you feel, think, and act in harmony with nature. You immerse yourself deeply in nature, in life, accepted for what it is, in the body, in sex, and in a healthy way of life.

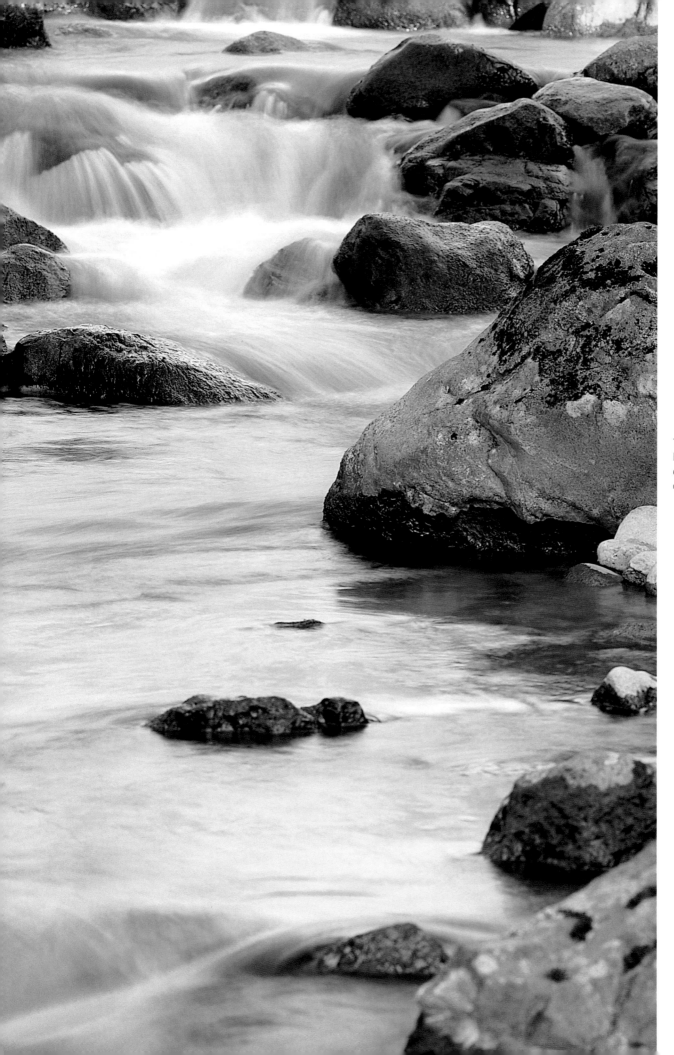

Tantra is like the bed of a river; its course is always changing.

TO BE AN INDIVIDUAL

It might surprise you to know that everyone with a big personality makes a show of it.

Etymologically, "personality" comes from "persona," which means "mask." The personality is, therefore, a collection of masks, of egos.

Individuality, on the other hand, is something entirely different; it is to know that you are unique, not by your ego but by your creation. There is no one else like you, and based on this premise, Tantra emphasizes individuality, not by separating you from others but making sure you don't blindly follow the flock, doing what you're told. With Tantra, the individual questions tradition and tests it for his or herself, bring their energy in order to leave the world a little better than how they found it.

Individuality also means that you are not divided inside—that you know

> If you cultivate energy, your vibration will grow bigger and align with the higher planes of existence.

what you feel and what you think. It doesn't mean you have to be superman or superwoman, just feel, think, and act from your roots.

Many people disregard their individuality and make it submissive. Submission does not allow you to express yourself and so you generate nothing. People are perceived by their wavelength, by their vibration, by what they emit. If you train in the art of Tantra and cultivate your energy, your vibration will grow bigger and align with the higher planes of existence, and you will find yourself connected

to its rhythm. It is like the drop of rain that falls into the ocean: once united, how can you tell the drop from the ocean? To fuse with the universe, to let your individuality take you back to it, is the goal, but to achieve this you must exercise the individual. Your life should be lived completely.

THE ORIGIN OF INTERNAL CONFLICTS: FEELING OR THINKING?

The physical body acts, the energetic takes prana, the astral feels, and the mental thinks. What happens then when we feel one thing but think the opposite? In that case, we have a conflict, which generates pain in the physical body (due to blocked energy) and later we may get sick. It is important to know that every human being has desires. You desire something in your heart, or in your mind, and then you look for a way to make it real, to have

THE INNER MAN AND WOMAN

The mystic union that Tantra seeks is realized first inside of ourselves, with the inner lover that each of us possess.

More than being man or woman, the human being is both, because it is born from androgyny. The male body produces estrogen just as the female body produces testosterone. **In a corner of every man is Shakti, the feminine energy, and in every woman we can find Shiva, the masculine.** *The tantric art consists of uniting the two polarities within each of us. Jesus also said: "When you convert two into one, and when you make the interior like the exterior and the exterior like the interior, and that at the top as that at the bottom, and when you convert the masculine to the feminine into one and the same . . . then you will enter into the Kingdom."*

We all have a yin and a yang, and this combination must be balanced so the inner lover emerges.

The man can awaken his feminine qualities—like sensitivity, perception, patience, relaxation, acceptance—and thus awaken his sexual energy more completely, rather than focused only in the genitals. The woman will awaken her masculine qualities—action, impulse, enthusiasm, impetus, wisdom, and the propulsion and expression of her thoughts—and sexually will take

initiative and enjoy the power of feeling how sensations go through her whole body as one.

Contact with the inner part of oneself is a bridge that will connect us to the deepest part of our being, and from this space we can discover our own light and share it.

The tantric relationship focuses on connecting those two poles of energy inside in order to then magnetize with the external partner—the electric and magnetic in full attraction. Discovering the feminine and masculine zones within ourselves is a challenge that will take us to the point of balance between genetic forces and those spiritual ones. To be clear, the chakras have a different polarity in each of us. **In women, the first chakra is negative and in men it is positive.** *The rest of the chakras are alternating: in women the second is positive and in men, negative, etc. Contact between the chakras, when they are already harmonized within our own bodies, will inevitably produce light; just as in a photograph, the positive follows the negative in order to reveal the visible. When the inner man and woman unite, the chakras polarize and are ready for the spiritual revelation, opening spaces in the consciousness to the deepest levels of bliss and unity.*

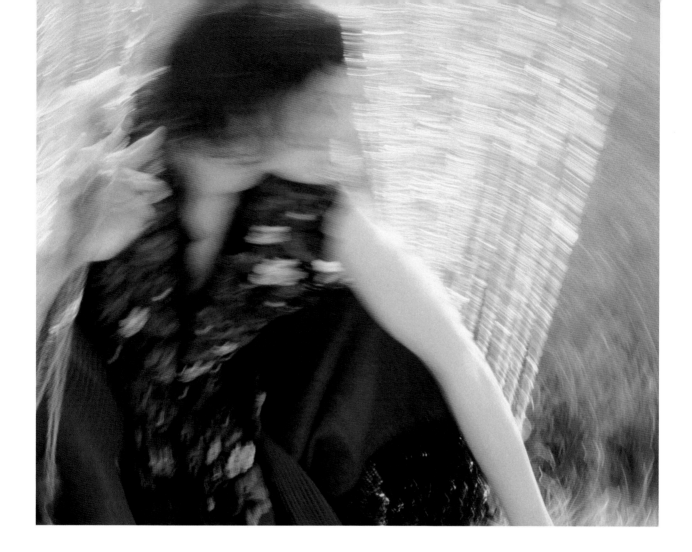

it materialize in the physical plane. When you achieve it, you get satisfaction, but if not, anxiety and anguish stay inside you.

There are people who find themselves in conflict because there is a disagreement between what they feel (that is, what comes from the heart) and what they think (what comes from the mind). But, what happens when you feel something deeply, something sensible, something full of feeling that will help you grow but your mind has a thousand and one arguments? This has happened to everyone.

In its negative phase, the mind is a receptacle full of repressions, fears, ideas, beliefs, false myths, negative thoughts, etc. When the mind is working badly, critically rather than creatively, it censures all that the heart wants to express. Obviously, the mind has positive functions. But suppose

that part is playing the role of censor or barrier; you will find yourself in a bind. A battle begins, not just between what you feel and what you think, but between the will to act on feelings and the mind's doubt to do it or not. For example, you love someone and you don't show it. You want to follow one path but your mind tells you the opposite. You have an emotion but you box it up with false morality. You want to have sex with someone but until your mind, you won't do it.

The world is full of repressed people, and a heart that represses its feelings is a spirit that can't laugh, leap, dance, and celebrate. The world is full of "serious" people because they think that being happy means being irresponsible. From this pursuit of seriousness have come many sicknesses and rigid personalities.

THE POWER OF THE GODDESS

In tantric tradition, the woman is the initiator of love, the bearer of life from her yoni to every cell. Whether as Shakti, Parvati, Kali, or Lakshmi, the woman is the luminous torch unveiling the mysteries of life, love, and sex.

The beauty of the women is as revered as her esoteric power, so physical beauty, sensuality, eroticism, and ardent passion are as important as sweetness, compassion, and sense of duty. Beauty is as much external as it is internal, since Tantra illustrates the soul of feminine divinity. Its aim is to awaken the Shakti of every woman.

The woman is the initiator of magical and mystical sexuality. She knows subconsciously all of the secrets, so it is only necessary to remember them. The woman should take an active role in sex, give power to the relationship, and provide the mystic power to the man.

It is also she who opens to door to the secrets of sexuality, although some Shaktis have forgotten this power through repression and the idea of sin that Puritanism has taught them.

Tantra liberates and gives consciousness. As Kaularahasya says: "The woman initiates through the same yoni from which the man was born, in a previous life. The woman initiates through the same breasts that fed the man, in a previous life. The woman initiates with the same mouth that, in another time, calmed the man. The woman is the supreme initiator of Tantra."

One should close their eyes and imagine the whole chain of women that have passed through the history of humanity so that the species continued, and lay worship to this noble act. If you observe the faces of women, you can see women with potential and others that are turned off, the repressed and the liberated. Each woman shows through her features her inner state. So the sexually active woman, orgasmic and mystic, will demonstrate happiness; she will be a radiant sun, will have fire in her gaze, dance in her hips, heat in her hands, willingness to act, and a meditative soul.

The woman that has her inner goddess very sensitive will want to dance, to enjoy, and to feel sexuality naturally in every moment, from looks to penetration of the lingam.

The yoni is worshiped as a giver of life and of sexual pleasure. The tantric woman is power, dance, sexual eroticism, and mystique. She is at once spiritual ecstasy and the pleasure of the skin. From Aphrodite, the goddess of love, Isis for the Egyptians, goddess of love, Priestess Suma of Babylon, Inanna, mother goddess of the Sumerians, Socrates' woman, Diotima, Mary Magdalene, the companion of Jesus, and so many others, woman has been seen as a stereotype of service and goodness, eros and sexuality.

Woman is a mystery of energies. The *Kama Sutra* says: "Not even those who are the object of her affection know the extent of a woman's capacity for love. This is due to the subtlety of a woman's love. Men rarely know women in their true beings, whether they love women or are indifferent to them, whether they delight in them or abandon them, not even when they take everything that they have."

Tantra immerses itself in feminine mystique and absorbs its energy in order to reach the divine. Within sexuality, the woman takes an active role and the man is passive. For example, in the position of Kali, she is on top of the man and drives him wild with the sensual movement of her hips.

FOUR TYPES OF WOMEN

The Kama Sutra classifies women in four types. The archetypes are:

1. The Lotus Woman:
Known as Padmini, her face is beautiful and her body delicate with soft skin. She has lovely breasts, bright eyes, and walks delicately. She speaks with a soft, musical voice and dresses well. Her yoni is perfumed and she likes to make love during the day.

2. The Elephant Woman:
Known as Hastini, small and strong, she walks slowly. She has rough, white skin, thick lips, and likes to eat in excess. Hungry for love, she likes to do it for long periods of time and at any moment. Her yoni is spicy.

3. The Art Woman:
Known as Chitrini, she is extremely beautiful and medium sized, with a thin waist, large breasts, and wide, sensual hips. She has a prominent yoni, with soft hair and the scent of sweet honey. She likes pleasure and knows the sixty-four tantric arts. She likes to make love at night.

4. The Oyster Woman:
Called Shankini, she has warm skin, a large body, small breasts, and a firm waist. Her head, hands, and feet are large. She has a rough voice, likes flowers and red clothing. She is hard, emotionally. Her yoni is always moist and has a salty flavor, with a lot of hair. She likes to make love mostly at night.

Worship of the yoni is found in many ancient cultures, as is the worship of the lingam, the erect masculine organ. It is seen as mysterious and the original source of procreation and spiritual power. "The Yoga Master should always pay homage to the feminine power, following the revelations of the Tantras. We should revere our mother, sisters, daughters, wife, and all women. During this type of worship, one should contemplate the essential unity of Wisdom and the Halves, the feminine and masculine principles." (Advayasiddhi)v

24

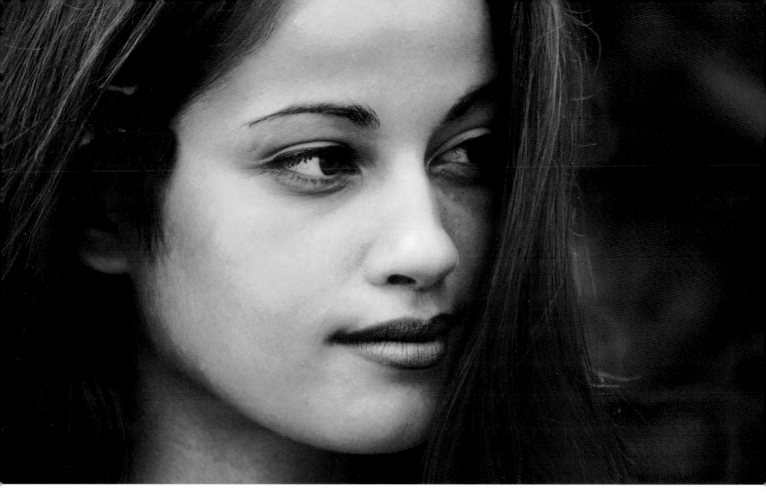

ADVICE FOR HARMONY IN A COUPLE

We need to maintain balance between giving and receiving in order to always have equilibrium. Remember the words of Erich Fromm: "Love is an art, not a thought."

Tantra is the art of fulfilling your role as lover and artist of your life. For this, I offer you some guidelines for a harmonious flow in the relationship with your partner.

▼ **YEILD.** We're not always right, so it is necessary to see the other point of view if there is a problem. "Problems are resolved with knowledge," says an Indian proverb. One day I learned an important lesson in regards to this principle, and it wasn't with a woman. I read in a book: "Give in and overcome." I understood it while driving my car on the highway. There were many cars around me going pretty fast, and the highway was rather narrow. Suddenly, I remembered the proverb

Tantra immerses itself in feminine mystique and absorbs its energy in order to reach the divine.

and I pulled over, letting the group of cars pass ahead of me. When I drove off, the whole highway was open for me to drive safely. What may seem like a loss, with time can result in a gain and greater comfort.

▼ **GIVE.** The gift is a ritual of adoration, not just for the individual woman but for what she represents, for the power she embodies. And the same goes for the man.

▼ **COMMUNICATION.** Beyond the verbal level, this is also the existential dialogue—what Tantra calls "Secret Language"—how to speak with the eyes, with the inner being, and the development of telepathy.

This is also what we call the language between the lingam and the yoni during maithuna.

▼ **SURPRISE.** An important factor to exploit novelty and vanquish the worst enemy: routine.

▼ **LIVE IN THE PRESENT.** Don't let the mind constantly project into the future; experience the here and now. Life doesn't sign long-term contracts. This also means you shouldn't think about lost years and get stuck in the past.

▼ **COMPANIONSHIP.** Support the occupations of both, be positive, and know that "he who doesn't live to serve, doesn't serve to live."

▼ **COMMUNAL PROJECTS.** Whether it is painting a picture together or watering and caring for a plant, whatever activity you can do together shares energy.

▼ **DO NOT ASSIGN BLAME.** Blame and fear have always been the invisible enemy to man, taught by the big institutions to maintain their power. Tantra tells you: "It's no one's fault!" Everything is an invention to make you feel guilty, as if you have to ask for-giveness. You shouldn't blame yourself for anything, but rather live your own "shared freedom." Guilt damages the fourth chakra and, as a consequence, makes it impossible to love.

The most important think you need to learn is to live freely. There is no temple more sacred than life; God doesn't close himself within four walls.

DANCE. Dance is an erotic and energetic instrument to help the movement of both energies find each other and fuse together. Life is not static.

Move with your partner (possibly naked) and feel your bodies and the way that bioenergy spreads from one to the other, creating a circle of power that nourishes you.

Remember that the stagnant and unnatural rots. Life is movement.

MASSAGES. An exchange of love where energy passes from one to the other helps to eliminate tension from the body and prepare it for maithuna, or simply leave it deeply relaxed. Read my book *The New Art of Massage* (Skyhorse Publishing) to find differ-ent techniques for massage, among them massage for couples.

INTIMACY. The sacred moments are those in which both people have an experience that no one else can touch: moments of ecstasy and expanded consciousness. But it is also important that each, separately, has moments of intimacy to be alone and connect with his or herself, as much as sharing secret moments and daily experiences, which are considered sacred.

TANTRIC PRINCIPLES

Although Tantra does not follow any principles or rules, we can glean (through direct experience) some guidelines to point you on the right path. This list should help you understand the tantric vision a little better:

▼ *Be simple and natural:* Don't get stuck on fashion or beauty stereotypes. There's no need to complicate or stick layers of ego on your personality.

▼ *Live spontaneously:* You will only achieve this by living from the heart. The mind calculates, projects, and separates you from the present. The spontaneous is like a child who always says what he feels.

▼ *Don't look for control, look for fluidity:* All control is unnatural. The biggest political control movements have fallen. Everything that one wants to control will escape sooner or later, like sand between fingers. It is better to adapt to the natural movement of things, just like the Ganges, which is never the same river.

▼ *Celebrate existence:* Be thankful each morning that you have another day to live and enjoy. Every day is different and you can make any of them special. You don't have to be sick to celebrate health, or lose your legs to value your ability to walk. It is a choice, a state of consciousness.

▼ *Live from freedom:* "Freedom" means doing what your heart tells you, and this means you won't be ruled by customs, repression, or conflictive people.

▼ *Raise your energy:* It is vitally important because it means you are working with your consciousness. When your energy is raised, your consciousness is as well, in each chakra. Energy is cultivated with practice.

▼ *Meditate:* Mediation, alone or with a partner, is the fountain that quenches the soul's thirst. When you meditate, the doors inside you open, generating better awareness, sensitivity, love, and a profound state of calm. You will see how to find the right meditation for the moment you are living. If you need to release tension from your body, first start with some active meditation; on the other hand, if you are looking for deeper peace, do some static, contemplative meditations.

▼ *Don't start conflicts between what you feel and what you think:* Feeling, thinking, and acting are daily movements for human beings. Obviously, when these are not in harmony you will feel a knot inside, a conflict: Which path to follow, what the heart feels or what the head thinks? How to act? Look deep, feel if it comes from your center, think whether it would harm others, and then act without remorse.

▼ *Be receptive and open to the universe:* We can live connected to the universe and thus be fluid and conscious, or disconnected, which produces feelings of separation, loneliness, and frustration. When you feel connected with your own consciousness and that of the cosmos, without intermediaries, you can feel the waves of energy, the ocean of consciousness, that is inside all of creation. This open state allows the heart to feel alive, healthy, playful, and vital. It has projects, enthusiasm, and feels supported. As Paulo Coelho says: "When you have a wish, the whole universe conspires to make it true."

▼ *Focus your mind on the present:* Almost all the Eastern spiritualities, like Zen, yoga, Tantra, Buddhism, and Sufism, highlight the importance of living in the present. Rationally we know that the past is gone and is unchangeable (and so it's useless to do anything) and the future is unreachable; so all that's left for us is the present. But the mind, like a restless monkey that goes from branch to branch, jumps from thought to thought. In a day, seventy thousand thoughts cross the mind. In this sense, meditation is the art of leaving the mind aside and perceiving the present, which signals to us which road our souls should take. It's important to be conscious that the present is eternity. If Life is eternal (Life with a capital L), then this eternity was there in the time of **Pitecantropus erectus** just as much as the time of Napoleon, and will continue forward, and so must be here now as well. There can be no space in time when the eternal did not exist. The key is to tune in to the here and now, discover the timeless present, and be conscious of eternity. The promise of eternal life after death is absurd because if it began when one dies, then it would have a beginning, and all that has a beginning has an end. For Tantra, eternal life is here and now.

▼ *Use your energy creatively:* You will get a lot of energy from practice and exercise. It's your responsibility to know what to do with this energy. You can bring it out in an artistic way, in your work, creating projects, loving, writing, or diving into yourself to do what you always wanted to. Creativity will flow in abundance. If the energy does not come out in a creative way, it can cause problems, pains, or dizziness. Keep an eye on your energy and look for the right path.

▼ *Sex is a manifestation of two trying to feel as one:* Sex is a phenomenon that can make you smell the perfume of unity. Sex has a spiritual and mystic connotation; on a small scale, it represents the universal laws of equilibrium of energies— the Sun and the Moon, winter and

EXERCISES FOR SINGLES

To call your soul mate, or the partner you want, you can do the following exercise: visualize a landscape, natural and sunny, clear river, trees, birds, and silver bridge with yourself at one end. Walk happily over the bridge to the other side and then wait for the image of your soul mate to appear.

It might appear in the first time, in a month, or when you are in the supermarket! The important part is that you are sending a message to the universe. Don't forget that everything you think can become reality; it all depends on the effort and intention you give.

summer, water and fire. In the same way, woman and man can experience a state of consciousness as one with creation. Tantric maithuna offers the way to reach this state of expanded consciousness.

▼ *Take care of the bindu, don't ejaculate:* When the man has an ejaculation, he loses the energy equivalent of half a liter of blood. Men have five liters, so half a liter of blood is a lot of fuel. Ejaculation also releases between three and five hundred sperm cells. After ejaculation, the man is drained and without desire. The blood leaves the lingam and it falls like a kite without wind. Tantra offers many techniques to avoid ejaculating and transmuting sexual energy (see chapter 9 for exercises and meditations). You can delay ejaculation for a long time, and thus the man can reach orgasmic sensations without loss of semen. Like blood, semen can't be made artificially. No laboratory can make these sacred components, so it's important to take care of them. It doesn't mean never ejaculate again; it depends how you feel. You can ejaculate once every ten times you have sex, for example. The art of not ejaculating and cultivating this energy depends on your skill, amount of practice, and constancy. Once you learn the trick it is not difficult, but it takes time. Many premature ejaculators benefit from

tantric techniques with no need for Viagra. The potential transmutation of ejaculation can make you a Buddha. When a man doesn't waste his semen, his personal vibration is strengthened, since one attracts what one emits. With a vibration of love, the body begins to generate energy and attraction. Purely energetically, not ejaculating gives the inner state a conscious connection with the energy of life. The concept of "brahmacharya" means "not ejaculating," "containing," and "alchemizing energy," so it doesn't mean chastity, not having sexual relations, it just means containing the bindu.

A very disciplined student of my course practiced every morning before work and commented that people told him that he seemed different, had a certain light and wellbeing. Certainly he was well because of the transmutation of energy. I told him it was because he carried his kundalini awake, and people noticed. What his friends saw was a point of light in movement; although they couldn't see it, they noticed. You can also reinforce your field of vibration if you follow the sadhana of Tantra, a constant practice. My interest, through conferences and seminars attended, is that everyone can have a tantric lifestyle with just a small change in attitude toward life. It is not just a way of sexuality. Although it teaches us to use sexual energy, this is just one step.

THE NEW TANTRIC BEATITUDES

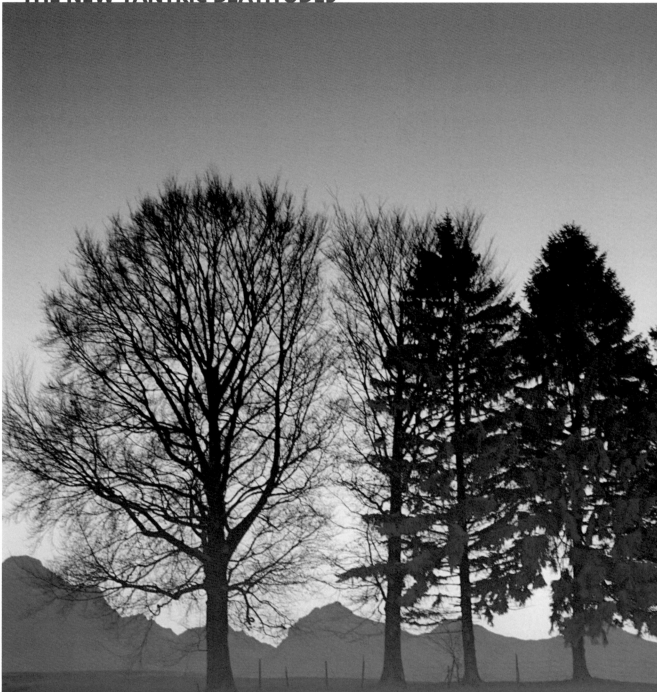

Blessed are they who are positive, for they will meet the sublime face of life. Blessed are they who don't criticize, for they will have creativity.

Blessed are they who are in love, for they are the only ones who are alive. Blessed are they who explode with happiness by breathing, for they will have life in abundance.

Blessed are they that reach orgasm, for the Big Bang is present in every moment.

Blessed are they who practice meditation, for they will vanquish death.

Blessed are they who love and care for their bodies, for this is the temple of the divine.

Blessed are they with open minds, for they will be free of false moral and sin.

Blessed are the mystics without dogma, for they will know supreme freedom.

Blessed are the lonely, for they can unite with others.

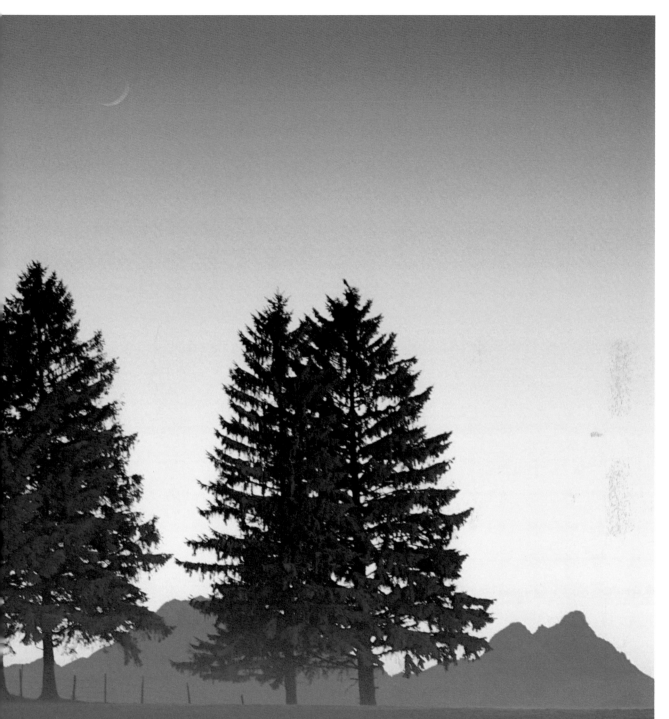

Blessed are they not driven by beliefs, for they will learn through experience.

Blessed are they with a healthy heart, for they will have innocence.

Blessed are they that understand what they feel, for they will be wise.

Blessed are they that act without interest, for their souls will fill with joy.

Blessed are they that are like children, for play will be the law of their life.

Blessed are they that fulfill their destiny, for they will live in peace.

Blessed are they that touch, smell, see, hear, and taste, for they will live without repression.

Blessed are they that are not afraid, for they will be protected by love.

Blessed are they that live without guilt, for the way will be open to them.

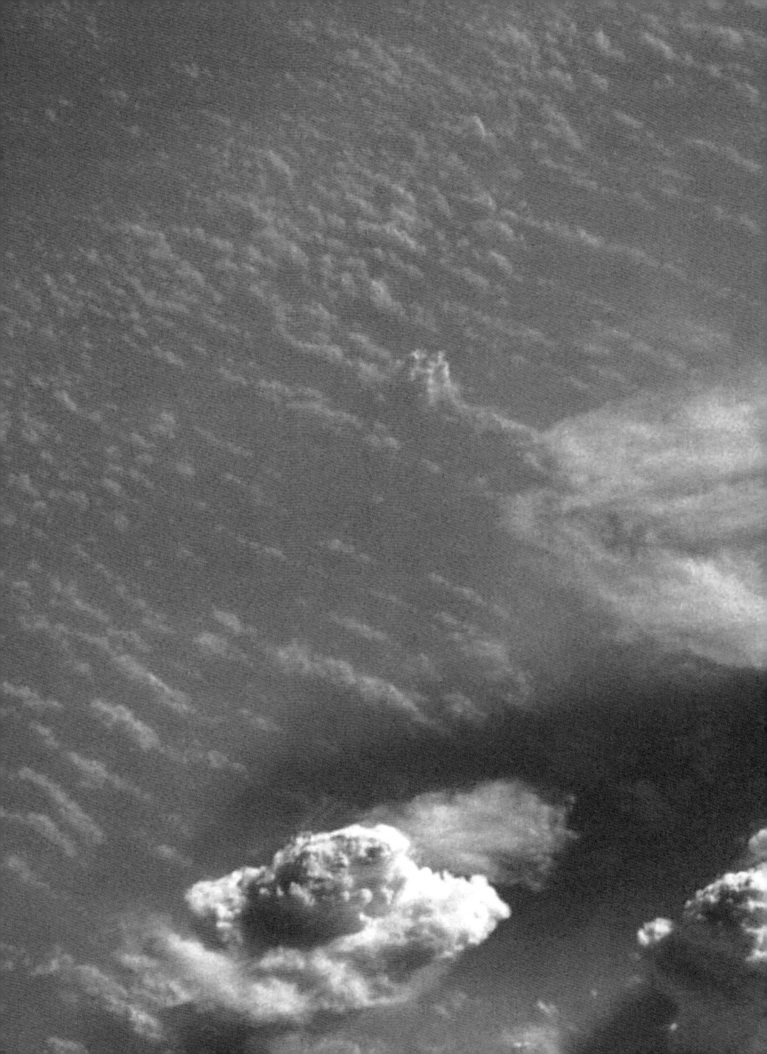

KUNDALINI
AND THE CHAKRAS

"The Kundalini is the motor of the human being.
The power of this energy
is the power of the Creation of the universe."

KUNDALINI:
The Psychosexual Energy

The energy that can carry man to his union with divinity is the "kundalini."

Located in the sacrosexual zone,

it can be awakened with various techniques.

The energy that can carry man to his union with divinity is the "kundalini." Located in the sacrosexual zone, it can be awakened with various techniques.

Eastern tradition affirms the existence of a sacred energy, called kundalini, that is found in all human beings in the first chakra, situated between the anus and the genitals.

From this chakra, once activated and developed, the kundalini—which has the form of a small serpent wound three and a half times around itself—emerges. It has been represented by this figure because it is the most meaningful; just as the serpent can rise up, the kundalini can rise through the central channel (sushumna) and elevate the consciousness and energy of the human through each of the chakras. The ultimate tantric quest is this act: to travel internally from the animal (the first three chakras: survival, sex, and food) to the human (fourth and fifth chakra: love and creating), to reach the sixth and seventh chakras (intuition and spiritual connection), the divine kingdom. Without exception, everyone has the ability to experience the inner journey to illumination, and that is why Tantra insists on energetic practice, sadhana.

The kundalini is sacred energy, which is why it is found in this zone. Through exercises in breathing, mantras, dances, meditation, sex, thoughts, and music, kundalini is awakened. However, before awakening and activating, purification of the body, mind, and emotions is essential, so that it doesn't find obstacles in its ascent. Said obstacles, such as fears, repressions, emotional conflicts, or muscle tightness, can be annoying and block energy as it rises.

When the kundalini energy begins to rise and activates each chakra progressively, these reveal all their qualities and talents that are normally inactive. That is why it is said that humans use only eight to ten percent of their capacity.

Once the kundalini is activated, the power of sex, self esteem, consciousness, creativity, and internal and spiritual vision are developed.

THE KUNDALINI AND ITS THREE STATES

1. Sleeping serpent
When it's in its latent state; in people that don't display much energy, that have a submissive, mild personality, and don't believe.

2. Serpent of wisdom
When it is activated by some means of sexual excitement and passes through some of the chakras without reaching the highest one, then sinks again. Every time a man ejaculates, the kundalini goes back to sleep, losing the desire, the electricity, and the magnetism of energy.

3. Dragon of living fire
The state in which the kundalini has risen and illuminated all the chakras to completely awaken the consciousness of the individual. It is moksha (spiritual liberation) and Samadhi (consciousness of the dissolution of Totality).

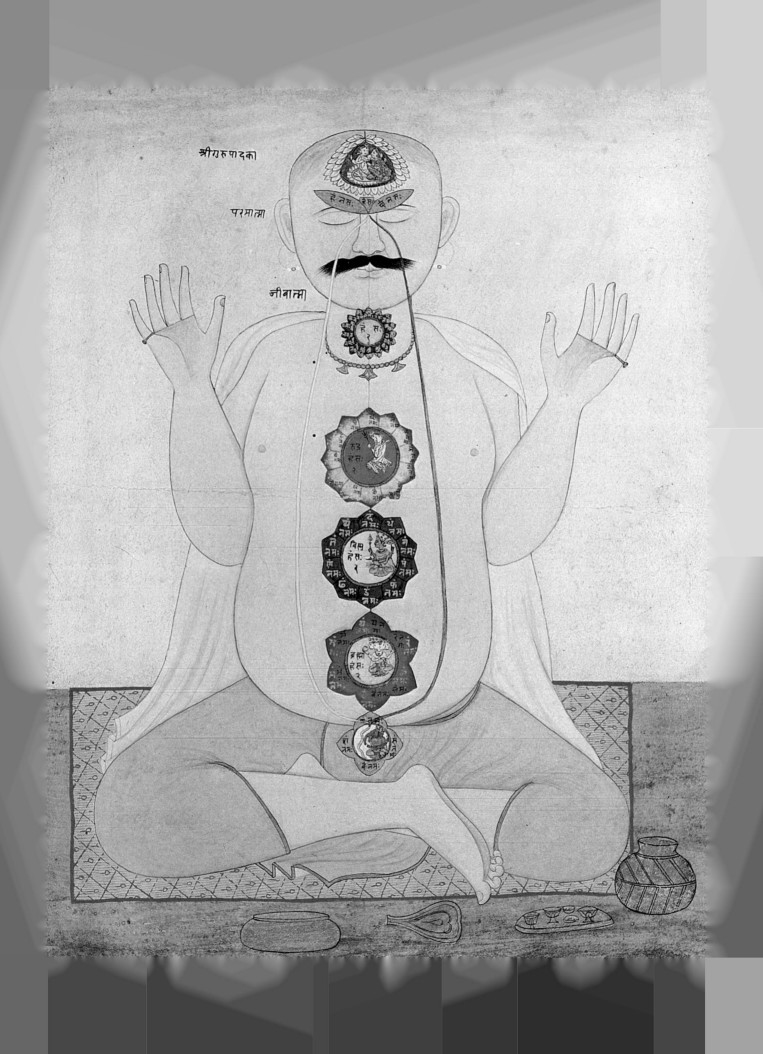

KNOWLEDGE AND HANDLING OF ENERGY

Energy needs conscious handling. Just like a car has the energy of the motor and fuel but needs someone to direct it, energy in all its forms in the body require conscious use to be most fruitful.

When the kundalini is freed, it is important to know what to do with it. We should have a creative focus to help it flow and give it a place to manifest itself without any roadblocks.

The first step consists of purification, which you can do through dietary changes (not a diet but oriented toward intelligent food choices, eating only what the body needs), practicing tantric tools (free dance, special breathing exercises, passive or active meditation, or conscious visualization of the chakras), or repeating a mantra (sounds with powers of spiritual vibration).

After purification, the kundalini energy will open the central channel to ascend. Let me be clear, this is not a quick process, it requires years of training. Each individual, according to his evolution, needs a certain amount of time. There are no formulas to predict when one's kundalini will ascend

Energy is one, but it has seven functions that, related to the chakras, indicate if the individual is in harmony or not.

completely; it is a conscious and individual process, although there are also powerful group exercises that elevate energy.

The planetary Shakti Kundalini is waking up in this era, as more and more people are drawn to practicing meditation, yoga, and internal sciences. The kundalini is the divine spark in the human body, and in traveling from the first chakra to the seventh it mixes with the spiritual energy that gives life, producing a regeneration in the cells, which fill with energy and light, as well as the spirit, which is nourished by consciousness, happiness and growth.

Tantra seeks to have the kundalini rise to the crown chakra, a sacred occurrence that the enlightened of the East and even Jesus have attempted. It can be observed in images, where they are surrounded by a golden aura around their heads; this is the sign

that energy has reached the crown chakra. This is also why ancient kings symbolically wore crowns.

For Tantra, he who wears his energy in the crown of his head is king of himself. It is a royal title that you can give to yourself—the universe will vouch for you!

Remember that kundalini energy can be freed spontaneously in people that are not necessarily on a spiritual path. Many who use drugs can experience a liberation of kundalini (although Tantra does not recommend this), as well as those who receive a hit in the sacral zone, during prolonged sex without orgasm, with meditation, in border states (fear, anger, deep sorrow), or during pregnancy.

Kundalini feels like waves that pass through the body, shaking or trembling, but also can be felt in the form of greater inspiration, and physical or spiritual strength.

THE TRUTH ABOUT SEXUAL ENERGY

"Energy" comes from "energon," which means "put into motion."

Energy is really all one, and although it has seven different functions, the only one that has been condemned is the sexual energy. But why? And by whom? We should know that when someone represses something,

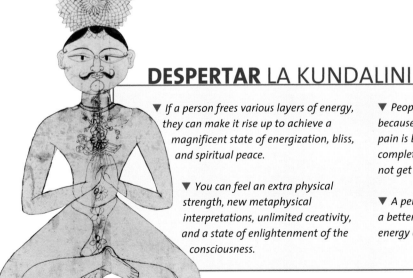

DESPERTAR LA KUNDALINI

▼ If a person frees various layers of energy, they can make it rise up to achieve a magnificent state of energization, bliss, and spiritual peace.

▼ You can feel an extra physical strength, new metaphysical interpretations, unlimited creativity, and a state of enlightenment of the consciousness.

▼ People with blockages might feel pain because they are not completely purified. All pain is blocked energy, so it is necessary to complete purification so that energy does not get clogged anywhere.

▼ A person who practices energetic work has a better chance of directing and channeling energy easily.

it's because they want to control it, and all that is repressed turns poisonous. It may surprise you to know that sexual repression emerged in several religions around the same time. Christianity, Judaism, and Islam condemn sex, falsely calling it "sin," word which means "to miss the mark." The truth is that sexual energy, when it is used for the transformation of spiritual energy, produces great power. Jesus (who had nothing to do with the postulates of the Catholic Church) said that if one has only an ounce of faith, he can say to a mountain "come," and the mountain will obey. The enormous creative and spiritual power of energy is what has forced institutions that want to control individuals to spread falsehoods about sexual desire.

Tantra, opening the mind, proposes getting to know that energy without being stuck in this point. You know it, you use it to reinforce your evolution and you allow the spiritual alchemy to happen within you. Evolution can be seen in two ways: individually or collectively. On one hand, humans evolve as a species, but on the other hand, when a person becomes conscious they experience an individual evolution. When sexual energy is focused tantrically for the evolution of the consciousness and not just for simple pleasure, it produces personal growth. And when people attract and repel each other, the same energy phenomenon emerges, not so much based on physical appearance but on the energy that each emits.

ACTIVATING ENERGY

Tantra is a manual on energy, the art and science of inner secrets. It knows that energy is one but it has seven functions that, related to the chakras, indicate if the individual is in harmony or not. When one function is weak or underdeveloped, the person begins to overload another chakra.

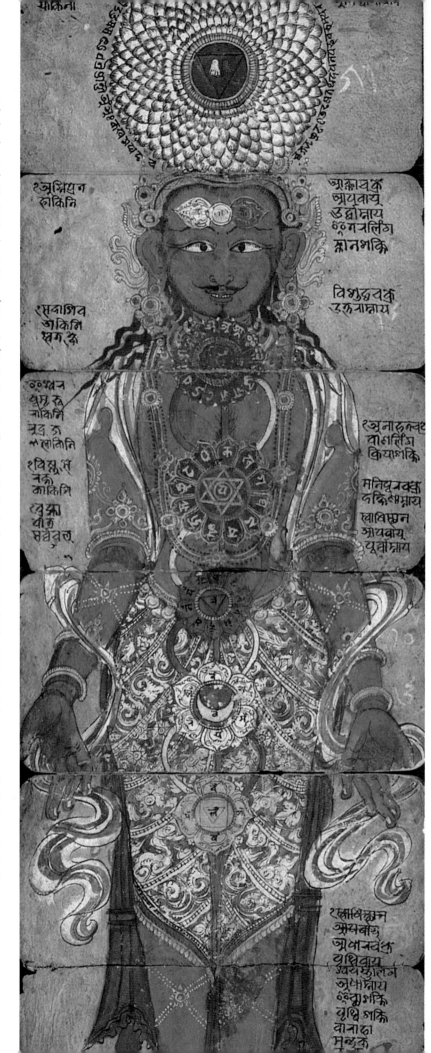

THE CHAKRAS POSSESS SEVEN BASIC DESIRES:

material survival; sexuality; food, love, and being loved; creativity; intuition; and spiritual connection.

35

Many obese people use their fat as armor, as if they had said: "I didn't put my energy into love, creativity, or spirituality, so I replaced it with food." Overeating often reflects an inability to balance the energy in its other functions because it can be done immediately, while sex requires seduction, attraction, art, etc. Love must be in contact with the self as well as the one to give it to.

The human body is naturally perfect, but it is up to the individual to care for it. Beauty, if it is truly subjective, is something that Tantra emphasizes. You should know that beauty comes not from your body, but from the interior, which reflects on the exterior. When you feel beautiful inside, you look beautiful on the outside. It is the magnetism of energy.

To balance the seven functions, it is important to be alert and conscious. Seeing yourself clearly is something that not only Tantra asks for. In the Temple of Delphi, in Greece, is the inscription: "Man, know yourself and you will know the universe and the Gods." Knowing yourself means diving into your inner world—feeling your energy, your inner state, the mechanisms of your actions, your ego, and your soul's desires.

Tantra activates energy to maximum expression; it activates and subsequently elevates it.

THE THREE MAIN NADIS

A nadi is a slender channel, like a hair in the energetic body, through which vital energy, or prana, circulates, feeding and vitalizing the physical body. Also called "meridians" by traditional Chinese medicine, there are about 72,000 nadis, and energy circulates through them as blood through veins.

The three main nadis have to do with the nostrils and the opposite pairings of the body. The right side of the body is masculine and the left, feminine; therefore the left nostril is feminine and lunar, and the right is masculine and solar. There are also two brain hemispheres, lungs, arms, genitals, kidneys, legs, and eyes. The organic balance is reflected in the human body.

The central channel is called sushumna, the right, pingala, and the left, ida. This nadis are cleaned through breathing exercises, or pranayamas, so that pranic energy feeds the chakras.

It is interesting to know that breathing is done through one nostril for about fifty minutes, then changes to the other. The body has its own thermostat to regulate its temperature and functions. When we breathe through the left nostril it stimulates the right hemisphere, useful for arts in general, like music, painting, writing, or holistic concepts. Breathing through the right nostril is useful for math, sports, sex, or physical activity. We breathe through both nostrils for intervals of only about ten minutes. Try putting a finger below each nostril and exhaling forcefully. You will notice that more air exits one, and in an hour, it will be reversed.

36

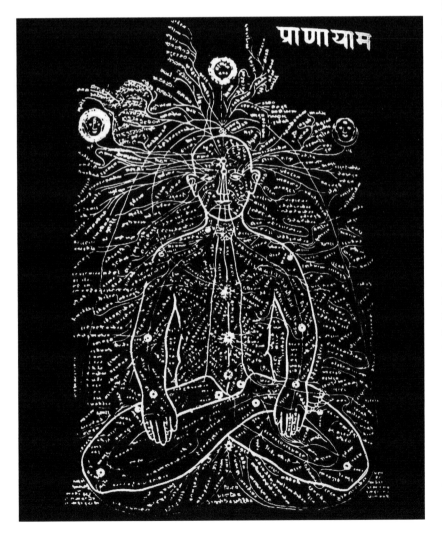

SYMPTOMS OF THE LIBERATION OF KUNDALINI

Kundalini acts differently in each person, since each has their own history, inner world, physical state, and development of energy, evident in their personality and daily attitude. Some of the symptoms a person may experience are:

▼ *Nosebleeds*

▼ *Yellowish skin tone, as the liver is cleaned*

▼ *Blackening of the big toenails, related to the pineal gland*

▼ *Involuntary shaking*

▼ *Intense emotions from blockages in the abdomen*

▼ *Seeing lights and colors, or other visual effects*

▼ *Change in physical state: you may appear rejuvenated or aged within a few days*

▼ *Disorientation, with yourself, others, or work in general*

▼ *Memory loss*

▼ *Moments of stupor or brilliance*

▼ *Signs of multiple personalities*

▼ *Unexplained illness*

▼ *Chills or hot flashes*

▼ *Eccentric behavior*

If you have these symptoms, you shouldn't think you're going crazy. You should just let the kundalini do its work by cleaning. Energy will rise to the top of the head and clean all the physical, energetic, emotional, and mental blockages on its way.

Let the kundalini grow upward in search of light, like a plant. The movements or waves of energy will help to produce liberation and improve your evolution. It's important to understand that during this cleaning process we should focus all our energy into it, without distractions or procrastination.

The journey of the kundalini is not a game; it is the mobilization of consciousness toward new and profound changes. This is when we should be most conscious and alert, continuing the work of purification with the certainty that it will be like the dawn after a dark night.

THE CHAKRAS

To understand the chakras as a symbol, imagine an invisible flute with seven holes that plays your personal music. Each hole represents a chakra, a confluence of metaphysical notes about human nature.

When the holes have energy, the music of your life flows harmoniously, but when they are blocked and "out of tune," the melody is wrong, just as a real flute if you don't play the right notes.

The cosmic flute that each of us has is in the spine, on the astral level. This is why the flute doesn't play music but rather energy, and the way it plays indicates if your life is in harmony or not.

The chakras are the wheels of energy, knowledge and potential that form the consciousness of the individual. They work through the kundalini (found in the first chakra), but also with the energy of the Sun and the air. The kundalini is psychosexual energy;

The nadis, called "meridians" in traditional Chinese medicine, number about 72,000 and circulate energy.

that which generates all of life's movement. There is no life in a human body without this energy. The kundalini flows along the central channel (sushumna) feeding the centers, the wheels of consciousness.

When energy is concentrated in a specific chakra, the person will have inclinations in their behavior based on the qualities of that chakra. The chakras generate seven basic desires,

as well as contain positive and negative personality traits. It all depends on whether they function well or have energy blockages, negative thoughts, sad emotions, or bad posture.

The first three chakras belong to the animal kingdom, since there is not much difference between a person and an animal in that they both want to survive, have sex, and eat. The next two are of the human kingdom; here a person loves, is loved, and can express themselves artistically. The last two (the third eye and the crown) belong to the divine kingdom and refer to the use of intuition, intellect and imagination, knowledge and spiritual desire. That is to say, we are animals turned to humans through love, with the potential to become conscious of our divine essence.

The consciousness of a person is affected when a chakra does not work correcetly. For example, if a person desires to love someone, but the love is unrequited, it will produce anxiety

37

THE 7 DESIRES

1. Muladhara Chakra	*Material desire, survival*
2. Swadisthana Chakra	*Sexual desire*
3. Manipura Chakra	*Desire for food*
4. Anahatta Chakra	*Desire to love*
5. Vishudda Chakra	*Desire to create and express oneself*
6. Ajna Chakra	*Desire for knowledge*
7. Sahasrara Chakra	*Spiritual desire*

and overload the food chakra, causing overeating or loss of appetite.

When we can't satisfy a desire immediately, we compensate by taking this energy to another. This causes an energetic disorder that affects the field of energy, and if it continues, can affect the function of a particular gland or organ.

If a person has more energy in the first chakra, their consciousness is in the material; they will talk about cars, houses, and material goods in general.

On the other hand, if they have their energy in the second, they will be focused on sex and see everything through a sexual lens.

If it is in the third, they will be the person that never stops thinking about food—after lunch, they'll start thinking about dinner.

If they have their energy in the fourth chakra (the heart), they will be a compassionate, loving, sweet, caring person, not in an egocentric way, but through natural goodness.

If the energy is in the fifth chakra, they will be creative, expressive, artistic, and soulful.

In the sixth chakra, or third eye, the person may be inclined to be intellectual, intuitive, or highly imaginative. With their inner perception, they will create a very sensitive field to intuit what will happen.

In the seventh chakra (in the top of the head), the person will be enlightened, connected consciously to the superior forces of the universe.

The spiritual destiny of every individual is to raise their energy from the two lower chakras to the top of the head. When they don't have harmony, there are problems in the different bodies. Energy is lowered and produces pains or illness in the physical body.

THE COMING AND GOING OF ENERGY

It's relatively simple to take in energy through tantric techniques. With an abundant flow of energy, the individual can empower and elevate their kundalini, initiating the process of spiritual transformation.

Energy has various entrances and exits. It enters primarily through the fontanelle on the top of the head, through the crown chakra. This first energy that comes from the Sun (cosmic prana) makes the heart beat and grants life. Energy also enters through the solar plexus and palms of the hands. All of the chakras receive prana energy.

The earth is another source of energy (apana) that rises through the soles of the feet. This is why it's very beneficial to walk barefoot on grass, earth, or the beach.

During seated meditation, the back is parallel to the earth's axis and receives mainly solar energy. When you lie on the ground, the chakras receive energy from the earth.

Energy enters naturally in these places for everyone, but through tantric techniques

THE SEVEN ENERGET
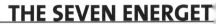

1. Physical body
The body that performs actions. It is also the densest of them all and visible to the human eye. Many people don't realize the wonders of the physical body: they don't know how many vertebrae they have, how many liters of blood, how many breaths per minute, how many miles of veins they have, etc.

The physical body is a perfect creation. Its natural state is healthy and flexible, but most people only experience this as children and grow rigid and unhealthy for lack of care.

2. Energetic body
The body that contains the 72,000 energetic channels called "nadis" or "meridians." Just as blood flows through the veins of the physical body, energy runs through the meridians of the energetic body. The ida, pingala, and sushama are found here, known as the lunar, solar, and central nadis. It is also important for acupuncture and shiatsu massage, which utilize twelve meridians (six yin and six yang) and the two extraordinary meridians that make up the microcosmic orbit. These are reserves of energy.

The function of this body is to maintain the physical with vital energy (prana) and absorb energy from the Sun and the earth (prana and apana).

3. Emotional or astral body
This body is ruled by feelings. The seven chakras and base of the psyche are found here, all connected to the glands and endocrine system of the physical body.

Each chakra has a function and generates a particular basic desire: material desire, sexual, food, emotional, creative, intuitive and intellectual, and the spiritual desire for divine unity.

When one of these desires is not in harmony or is unsatisfied, energy overloads another chakra and causes an imbalance. For example, someone who wants to buy a house (material desire), but has to wait, will eat out of anxiety (desire for food).

Every day we see how one chakra is overloaded because the desire of another cannot be satisfied.

4. Mental body

Here are the thoughts, ideas, projections of the future or memories of the past, calculations, intellect, beliefs, etc. The mind, driven by thought, is a great mystery with much potential to develop. The mental body, like all of them, varies from one person to another. There have been wars and people have killed others because of differing ideas. The mind is an impediment to harmonious relations from the soul and consciousness, because everyone has beliefs that impede their consciousness. A mind used badly distances people because it divides and isolates people from their centers. The emotional body is run by feelings and the mental by thought, and how many times have you felt one thing and thought another contrary thing? If we think differently than we feel, the action won't happen. The individual needs to think and feel in harmony in order to act successfully. If we feel A and think B, there is an inner conflict and the conflict of energies between bodies generates pain and illness. With Tantra we reestablish the flow of energy, harmonize it, balance the bodies, and mobilize the psyche.

The mind has been filled with unnatural beliefs; the spirit has been burdened with blame and suffering and we flagellate the body in the name of the spirit. Now we need to empty ourselves, and Tantra allows for a contact that silences the mind, opens the heart and emotion, and relaxes the body, increasing vital energy.

5. Spiritual body

This is the plane of perception. As long as there are so many disputes between the other bodies (between feeling and thinking), the spirit cannot flourish and develops very slowly, as do the next two bodies.

We put too much emphasis on satisfying the mind's needs, so the spiritual body opens little by little, to a large field of perceptions and abilities.

The spirit is the shell of the soul, and the spiritual body, through tantric practices, deep meditation, or simply sleeping, gains expression that manifests as new octaves of interior knowledge.

6. Cosmic body

This is a much higher plane, although attainable. In fact, these final three bodies must be created. They are like seeds we need to care for so they flourish in the soul.

The cosmic body fuses the individual to divinity, allowing access to the real, holistic world, where boundaries disappear. There is no "here" or "there," the consciousness takes it all as One.

7. Nirvana

In this stage, the ordinary I disappears into the infinite consciousness. It is enlightenment, the return to home. The divine play (lilah) is projected into eternity. On this plane, the apprenticeship has ended. In the words of Jesus: "My Father and I are one and the same."

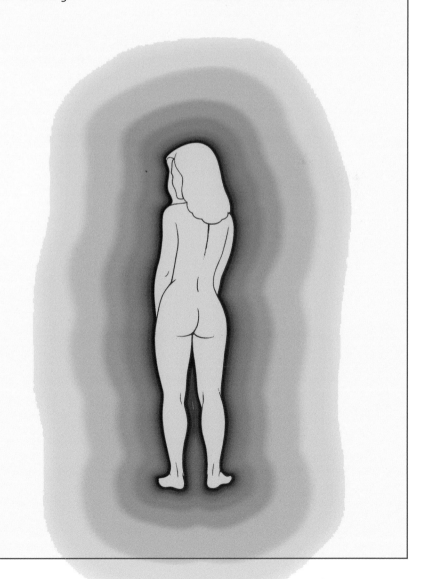

THE CHAKRAS

FIRST CHAKRA: *Root*
The right to have

This chakra expresses the right to survival. This includes money, property, and all worldly possessions. The tantric way emphasizes the stimulation of the first chakra with dance, massage, breathing, and music to activate the kundalini. In massage, we use specific techniques to empower and align this chakra.

Name: *Muladhara*
Element: *Earth*
Influential signs: *Taurus, Virgo, and Capricorn*
Personality: *Earthly*
Plexus: *Coccyx*
Location: *Base of the spine, between anus and genitals*
Endocrine gland: *Testicles or ovaries*
Desire produced: *Survival, comfort, economic wellbeing, and relation to the earth*
Aim of the chakra: *Prosperity, abundance, comfortable life, and economic stability*

Symptoms of balance: *Sure of oneself, controls desire*
Symptoms of imbalance: *Egotism, depression, instability, inability to save money, timidity, easily distracted, the feeling of escaping or not having concrete things, inability to enjoy*
Symptoms of overuse: *Attachment to security, fear of any change, obsession with material goods, overweight, anxiety from eating*

Expression in the body: *Hemorrhoids, sciatica, prostate, constipation, knee problems, poor circulation in legs, bone problems*
Color: *Intense red*
Gems: *Garnet, black tourmaline, red stones*

SECOND CHAKRA: *Sexual*
The right to feel

This chakra manifests as free expression of sensitivity, sensuality, and sexuality. It is the driving chakra of the most important energetic function: sexuality.

Name: *Swadisthana*
Element: *Water*
Influential signs: *Cancer, Scorpio, and Pisces*
Personality: *Aquatic, mobile, fickle*
Plexus: *Spleen*
Location: *Approximately eight centimeters below the navel*
Endocrine gland: *Suprarenal*
Desire produced: *Sexual, unity of opposites: Yin and Yang, Shiva and Shakti, masculine and feminine*
Aim of the chakra: *Pleasure, conquest, opening and controlling of sexual energy*

Symptoms of balance: *Resistence, patience, confidence, wisdom about sexual desire; "Kama," desire, "Sutra," wisdom*
Symptoms of imbalance: *Anxiety, fear, rigidity, cold, impotence, instability, bottling of emotions.Lack of sensitivity, talking unnecessarily (the tongue is connected to the sexual center, this is why when someone kisses with tongue it awakens sexual energy).*
   Many people talk too much because they don't have a good sex life and discharge energy by talking.
Symptoms of overuse: *Sex addiction, anxiety of pleasure, extreme sexual desire, possessiveness, jealousy, close mindedness, inability to self satisfy, dependency on another*

Expression in the body: *Kidneys and bladder, prostate, sexual organs*
Color: *Bright orange*
Gems: *Coral, orange stone*

THIRD CHAKRA: *Alimentary, strong emotions*
The right to work

This chakra is related to will power, vitality, personal power, and self-esteem. It receives all of the lower emotions (fear, anger, worry, and anxiety) and they remain trapped in the organs, affecting their function.

Name: *Manipura*
Element: *Fire*
Influential signs: *Aries, Leo, and Sagittarius*
Personality: *Passionate and energetic*
Plexus: *Solar*
Location: *In the mouth of the stomach*
Endocrine gland: *Pancreas*
Desire produced: *Alimentary*
Aim of the chakra: *Provide vitality, unbreakable will power, inner power, motivation to act.*

Symptoms of balance: *Personal power, determination, just actions*
Symptoms of imbalance: *Doubt, timidity, low energy, fatigue, digestive problems, submission, obesity*
Symptoms of overuse: *Mood swings, desire to dominate others, anger and frequent outbursts, ulcers*

Expression in the body: *Heart and respiratory problems, arterial hypertension*
Color: *Green*
Gems: *Green or pink quartz, emerald*

FOURTH CHAKRA: *Heart*
The right to love and be loved

This chakra is linked to everything emotional. It represents the desire for emotional unity, love, and fraternity. Manifested in affection, compassion, love, tenderness, and solidarity.

Name: Anahatta
Element: Air
Influential signs: Gemini, Libra, and Aquarius
Personality: Loving, sensitive, solitary
Plexus: Cardiac
Location: In the center of the chest
Endocrine gland: Thymus
Desire produced: To love and be loved
Aim of the chakra: Balance in relationships, strong bonds with others and oneself

Symptoms of balance: Compassion, acceptance of reality, emotional openness
Symptoms of imbalance: Instability, emotionally closed, loneliness, sadness and melancholy, passivity, low self-esteem, sunken chest, shallow breathing
Symptoms of overuse: Situations that depend on others, excessive clinginess or detachment

Somatiza en el cuerpo: Problemas cardÌacos y respiratorios, hipertensiÛn arterial.
Color: Verde vida.
Gemas: Cuarzo verde, esmeralda y cuarzo rosa.

FIFTH CHAKRA: Throat
The right to speak and express oneself

This chakra provides the capacity for communication, artistic expression, and truth. One can communicate, express, and create in tune with universal creation as long as they are balanced and in harmony.

Name: Vishudda
Element: Ether
Personality: Mobile
Plexus: Larynx
Location: In the throat
Endocrine gland: Thyroid
Desire produced: To communicate, express oneself
Aim of the chakra: Express oneself to others in harmony with the interior, creative use of energy

Symptoms of balance: Artistic, creative development (whatever the activity), spiritual elevation
Symptoms of imbalance: Stagnancy, obsession, repression of what you want to say, inability to say it, creative block; throat irritation, loss of voice, wry neck, shoulder stiffness
Symptoms of overuse: Talk a lot and say little, shouting, verbal diarrhea

Expression in the body: Throat pain, voice problems, hipo- or hyperthyroidism, flu
Color: Lavender blue
Gems: Aquamarine, turquoise

SIXTH CHAKRA: Brow
The right to intuit

This chakra is in charge of the ability to clearly perceive things that happen through intuition, which is a function of the soul. It also exercises imagination and intellect. Once activated, it awakens extrasensory abilities.

Name: Ajna
Element: Thought
Personality: Intuitive, imaginative
Plexus: Frontal
Location: Between the eyebrows
Endocrine gland: Pituitary
Desire produced: Power through inner knowledge
Aim of the chakra: Grant clear vision of events, know through intuition, which means "to see inside"; awaken the sixth sense, which is internal.

Symptoms of balance: Psychic abilities, lucid intellect, extrasensory perception
Symptoms of imbalance: Insensitivity, inability to imagine new ideas or use intuition, incredulity of dreams or revelations; lack of ability to visualize or project. Intellectual stagnancy, isolation

Symptoms of overuse: Paranoid fantasies, nightmares, hallucinations

Expression in the body: Headaches, confused thoughts
Color: White
Gems: Lapis lazuli, white quartz

SEVENTH CHAKRA: Crown
The right to Know

The lotus flower on the top of the head that receives divine energy and the gift of life. A spiritual sun that connects the individual to God. It is the extinction of duality because when it awakens, the consciousness fuses with divinity.

Name: Sahasrara
Element: Light
Personality: Crosses boundaries of the personal, uniting oneself with the spiritual
Plexus: Crown
Location: Top of the head
Endocrine gland: Pineal
Desire produced: Spirituality, mystic union
Aim of the chakra: Expand the consciousness

Symptoms of balance: Cosmic consciousness, enlightenment, inspiration, seeing on a higher level
Symptoms of imbalance: Depression, madness, psychosis, confusion, slow mindedness, worry, rigidity of personal beliefs, close mindedness
Symptoms of overuse: People who believe they know everything or always want to be right; spiritual and intellectual elitism; awakening of the most dangerous personal ego; isolation, disassociation

Expression in the body: Tumors, pressure on the skull
Color: Violet
Gems: Amethyst, diamond, white quartz

it is possible to increase the daily energetic quota, and greater energy means greater creativity.

When energy is absorbed but not used creatively, it comes out negatively. Energy is lost in arguments, rage, worries, and low emotions, through uncontrolled sexual activity, or fear. If you lose energy you will feel down, so maintain it and increase it; treasure its level of vibration.

We all absorb energy naturally, but with tantric techniques we can increase our daily energetic quota. And more energy means more creativity.

ENERGY AND THOUGHT

One energetic law says: "Energy follows thought." That is to say that, as you think, so will be your level of energetic vibration. For example, if a person is thinking in complaints, from the feeling of "I can't," this will be the consequence. If you think you will lose, so it will be; if you think you will achieve it, you will. Many people distrust this principle, blaming their situation on destiny or others. Human beings don't know their power: that of free will, with which they can complete everything they have in mind. Thought is not vain, it is the most subtle form of energy.

A repeated thought generates an idea; an idea, if it persists, will form a belief; if this belief is unnatural or negative, with time it will develop into illness (almost all illnesses originate in thoughts that are incompatible with the vibration of life). If you take note of the tides of daily thoughts that you have, you will have a visible example of what's in your head, which is what makes your future. All of the beliefs, plans, worries, and ideas form your life.

Modern man uses his mind all the time, so this inner space cannot fill with silence. Imagine that the engine of your car runs continuously when you aren't using it: with time, it will break down. With tantric meditations, you can develop the power to "turn on" and "turn off" your mind.

On the sexual plane, the mind is the greatest organ. When it focuses its energy on sex, it becomes all fantasy and imagination, which can take two paths. To the Right, you imagine the sex act. Thinking of someone can awaken sexual energy and desire for their body, as well as their energy.

THE CHAKRA TEST

Circle the letter you most identify with. These aspects have to do with each of the chakras and will show you where you have the majority of consciousness and where you have to work more. The letter "A" corresponds with the first chakra, "B" with the second, and so on.

FEARS
- a. Fear of physical harm and death
- b. Fear of being excluded
- c. Fear of rejection and dissatisfaction
- d. Fear of loss
- e. Fear of change
- f. Fear of responding spontaneously (doubt)
- g. Fear of chaos

COLORS
- a. Red
- b. Orange
- c. Yellow
- d. Green
- e. Blue
- f. White
- g. Violet

LOVE AND SEX
- a. He/she is so cute! I want to eat him/her up!
- b. We were made for each other!
- c. He/she is so confident! I'm proud! He/she suits me!
- d. My heart is leaping from my chest! I am fulfilled!
- e. I have a lump in my throat! He/she leaves me speechless!
- f. I'm losing my head! He/she dazzles me!
- g. He/she has magic, a radiant aura! I feel devotion!

WHAT ASPECT OF YOURSELF DO YOU WANT TO FIX OR IMPROVE?
- a. Economic situation
- b. Sex life
- c. Diet and self-esteem
- d. Feeling of abundance to love and be loved
- e. Lack of creativity and expression
- f. Inability to see things clearly
- g. Feeling of disconnect with the universe and life

WHICH PART OF YOUR BODY DO YOU LIKE MOST, AND WHICH THE LEAST?
- a. Legs, knees and butt
- b. Hips and sexual area
- c. Abdomen, abdominals, and waist
- d. Chest, breasts
- e. Neck, teeth, and mouth
- f. Eyes and gaze
- g. Head and hair

Observe which aspects you marked and work internally through energetic practice described in the following chapters.

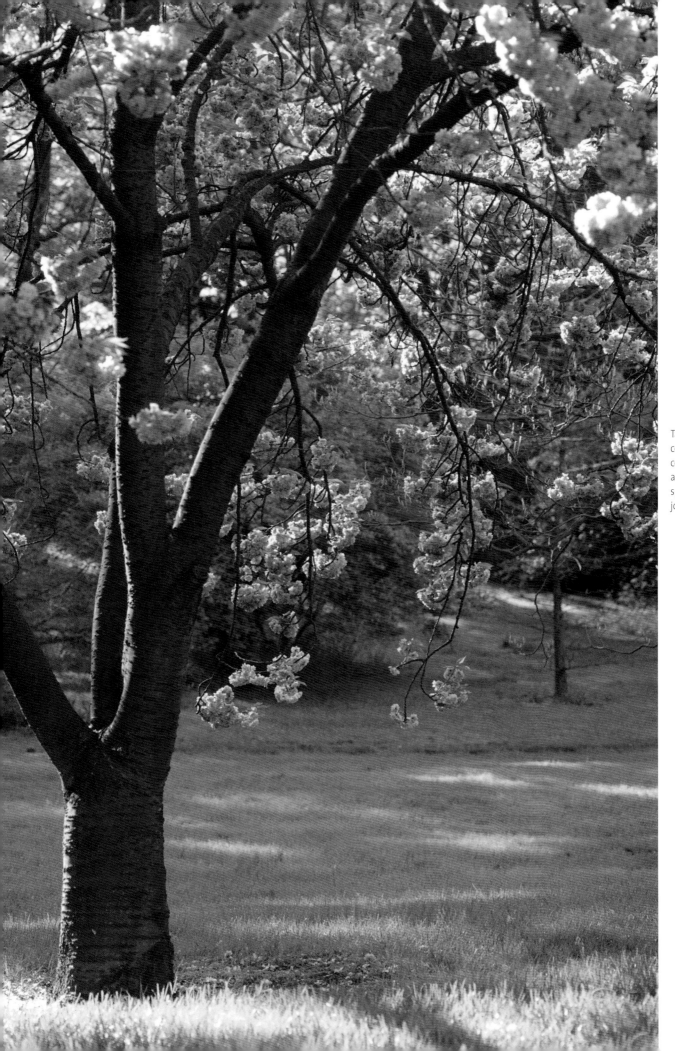

Tantra is a complete path: it combines roots and fruit, sex and spirit, silence and joy.

On the other mental path, you arrive at pathology (morbid curiosity, voyeurism, and many other forms of sexuality), and although Tantra doesn't condemn this, it does differentiate it from the sublime because these feelings to not allow the elevation of energy (they awaken energy only in the genitals).

Therefore, the mind needs to rest. With the techniques of this book, you will learn the secret to disconnecting the mental flow, entering spaces of your being where there is only consciousness—a journey beyond the mind.

MAGIC ENERGY: A DOUBLE-EDGED SWORD

Tantra produces magic because all energetic practice is really a magical practice. However, although Tantra considers magic the basis of creation (it uses sex to awaken spiritual power), it also has a scientific, artistic, and spiritual lens. As Richard Bach says in *Bridge Across Forever:* "We are not dust, but Magic."

The magical is related to life in all its dimensions: there is magic in the leap of a frog, the movement of the planets, the beat of a heart, or breathing.

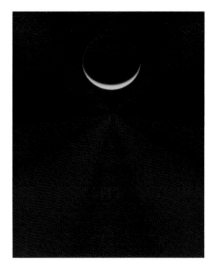

Magic is just around the corner and with the tantric union of breathing and imagination you can create something on a subtler plane than the physical. It works with the body and sex, but also with the higher planes, such as the astral, which is our second home.

To understand this ability, remember what the Bible says: "And that which I most feared, came to pass." When one is afraid that something will happen, it ends up happening, not because you cause it but because the energy you give to this thought makes it bigger and stronger, like a snowball. Not in vain, "energy follows thought."

This polarity is negative magic, which is self-destructive. White magic, on the other hand, is a symbol of power for Tantra, the connection with the higher luminous zones of existence. If evolution is an individual journey, we are not alone; the air is full of "presences." Many advanced followers and masters of Tantra create, with their inner power, the possibility of higher forms of spiritual nature.

In maithuna, the tantric sexual ritual, the couple can connect through the same thought and emotion to create magical force. They can focus the energetic flow into the magic river of existence to obtain something specific.

The power of magic is present in Tantra like the power of the invisible. In fact, love is the magical energy that moves all functions, from the cellular to the spiritual. Love is an incantation.

As Osho says: "You meditate because you are not living in love; when love emerges there is no need for meditation"; "Meditate lovingly and love meditatively." Meditation, the inner search, the diving into ones own inner world, serves to shed personal layers and armor to contact the love we have inside, for which we were created, and which is the only magical power on Earth.

ENERGY AND EMOTIONS

Emotions are also energetic movements. A repeated emotion forms a feeling, and a chain of feelings in the astral body determines the circulation of energy through the chakras.

There are **negative** or low emotions, which cause a short circuit in the animal chakras. Arguments, anger, worry, and fear affect the liver, spleen, kidneys, stomach, and the three basic chakras. There are also **higher** emotions—like love, tenderness, companionship, happiness, or enthusiasm—that activate the human and divine chakras. The center of the chest, the throat, the third eye, and the crown chakras are activated by luminous and expansive energy.

Emotions have to run their natural course and be expressed, since what you express is the emotional energy leaving the spirit. When emotions aren't expressed, it causes blockages on various levels. With dance, massage, special breathing, and meditation, we produce a constant movement of emotions—a torrent of sensations that allow us to know and observe the inner world.

In the deepest inner states, all emotion will cease and an emptiness will remain that includes all; the mystic space, free of bonds but full of joy and peace, that is the goal of tantric practice. It is not unreachable for modern man if he unites the spiritual with the quotidian, survival and material comfort with meditation.

Sooner or later, everyone will end up swimming in the waters of spiritual emotion; the experience of returning to the state of light and consciousness.

With Tantra, we don't repress emotions.

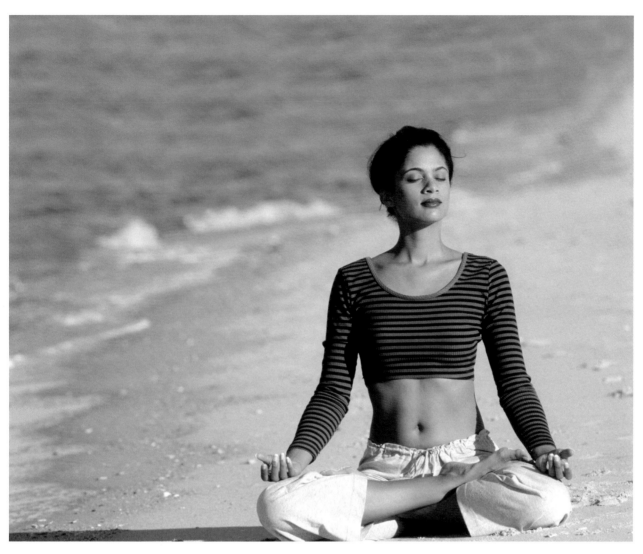

45

Meditation serves to shed personal layers and armor to contact the love we have inside, for which we were created.

When you are in tune with the heart of life, you enter a connection with the heart of God; from there, your individual heart fills with magic. Magic is a state of enchantment where the boundaries of the mind, of logic, of the visible and invisible, dissolve, generating the divine presence in your existence.

Magic can be a double-edged sword for he who increases his energy and doesn't cultivate consciousness, so it is necessary to elevate both to equal levels. To quote Richard Bach once more: "Love is like two balloons that float up together into the sky." Interpreting this phrase metaphysically, what Bach proposes is that the le-

vel of evolution and that of the consciousness tend to be similar, since if one rises more than the other, the distance between partners increases.

Rituals can serve to strengthen the energy and consciousness in

couples, by broadening their vibratory field, where energy crosses from one body to the other and mix, creating the sacred "tantric circle," a "feedback" of energy and light in the astral plane. These energies should be carefully focused in one aspect; they can't be left adrift. It is vital to have a goal ahead of time to know where the mobilized energy will go. For example, you can aspire to more love in the couple, completion of a project, the visualization of a dream house, better spiritual connection, increased economic gain, etc.

Magic can make you a being conscious of your light, of your inner power, and your divine origin, that God is not outside, but inside of you. You are ready to act because the power spilling from you is so strong; your life is a wonder.

When magic manifests itself, ego disappears, and only consciousness of love remains. This level of consciousness is God.

HANDLING AND TRANSMUTATION OF ENERGY

Tantra emphasizes using energy intelligently.

To live an existence full of negative thoughts and emotions, without energetic practices, causes you to lose most of your energy. Physical activity without recycling does as well. Take, for example, an elementary teacher that takes care of lots of children, or an employee that serves lots of people daily: contact with so many people is dangerous for physical and energetic health because you need to have a very strong vibratory field.

> A follower of Tantra should protect the energy they develop, just as someone who grows wheat protects it from frost and pests.

It is necessary to protect the energy you develop, just as someone who grows wheat protects his seeds from frost and pests.

Being attentive to people around us without letting them "suck" our energy is a practice of consciousness.

It's important to know this, since when you elevate energy, other people unconsciously perceive this and absorb it from you.

The tantric individual cares for their energy like their greatest treasure.

HOW TO BRING ENERGY TO THE CHAKRAS

Tantra teaches all aspects related to the growth of the individual. It knows that the human "mold" is equal in all because all of us have seven chakras; what differentiates us is the development and openness of each one. The singularity of people is determined by their culture, personality, appearance, inner world, beliefs, etc. The human essence, however, is always the same. The aim is to consciously stimulate the chakras for the development of the person.

The transformation of the chakras is achieved through constant practice. It consists mainly of a combination of techniques where breathing is the pillar of storing prana: dances to move it, and visualization and meditation to awaken each chakra.

The chakras receive energy and then externalize it in different ways, such as creativity, inspiration,

46

THE DIFFERENT ENERGIES OF THE DAY

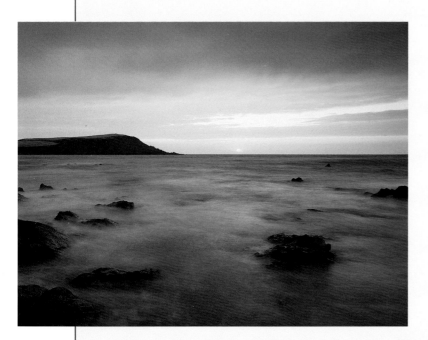

Sattva, Rajas, and Tamas
Energy has three different functions each day: it is "sattvic" (pure) from 4 a.m. until noon; "rajasic" (active) from noon to 8 p.m.; and "tamasic" (inactive) from 8 p.m. to 4 a.m.

Nature has energetic cycles (like the movement of the planets) that we can take advantage of to meditate in the morning, work later, and rest last. It is inconvenient to alter these rhythms. People who work at night, for example, have countless problems, from premature aging (at night there is no solar prana to nourish the cells) to memory loss.

According to Tantra, you should not have sex after two at night because the energy circulating at this time is not good for spiritual development.

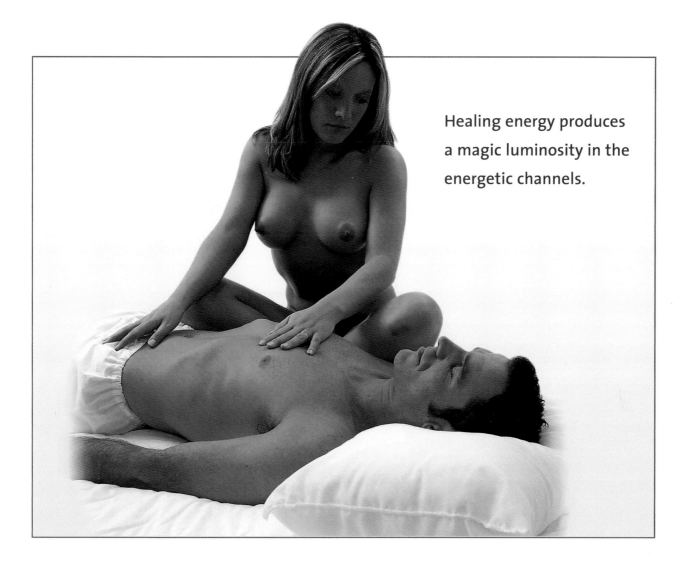

Healing energy produces a magic luminosity in the energetic channels.

flashes of symbols or new ideas, a greater capacity for love, an increase in sexuality, and a greater consciousness of oneself and ones extrasensory powers (telepathy, clairvoyance or "seeing clearly," memories of other lives, premonitions of the future, and symbolic dreams).

The techniques in the practice section of the book will orient you on how to activate the chakras.

THE ATTACK ON THE FOURTH CHAKRA

The individual has been broken up and divided throughout centuries.

In the dichotomy of having to choose—between good and bad, moral and immoral, decent and indecent—we have fallen into the grip of the worst enemy: guilt.

Many times one does things subconsciously, while sleeping or automatically. In the name of tradition, man has become stupid, without spontaneity or effervescence. Have you ever stopped to think that when you attend Christian mass, you have to hit your chest three times and repeat "through my fault, through my fault, through my fault"? Did you know you are closing the fourth chakra (which Jesus said should be opened)?

Did you know that if you feel guilty, the fourth chakra (in the center of the chest) closes and you cannot love? But in reality, it's even worse, since a closed chest not only prevents you from loving out of guilt, but also prevents you from experiencing enjoyment. If you eat good food but can't

stop feeling guilty because there are hungry children in the world, you won't enjoy it. Don't believe you are safe from this, because the idea of guilt is hidden in a very deep corner of the subconscious. In this aspect, the Church has created a rat in the mind and heart of humans. For what? Because if you feel guilty all the time, you will need an "intermediary" to "save" you. Think about it: if God is all around, why not talk to Him in the shade of a quiet tree?

Tantra must complete a deep cleaning of the chakras, especially the fourth, because it is a way of love and love comes from the fourth chakra. Without the openness of the fourth chakra, you cannot live happily as children do, innocent, dynamic, and joyful.

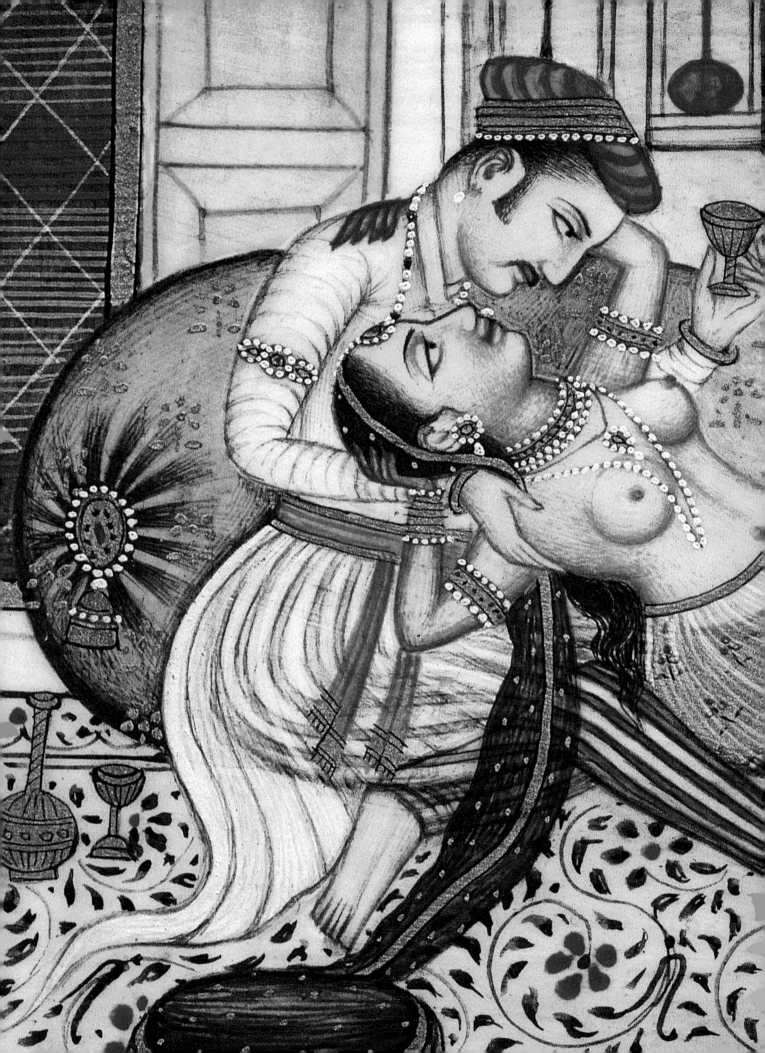

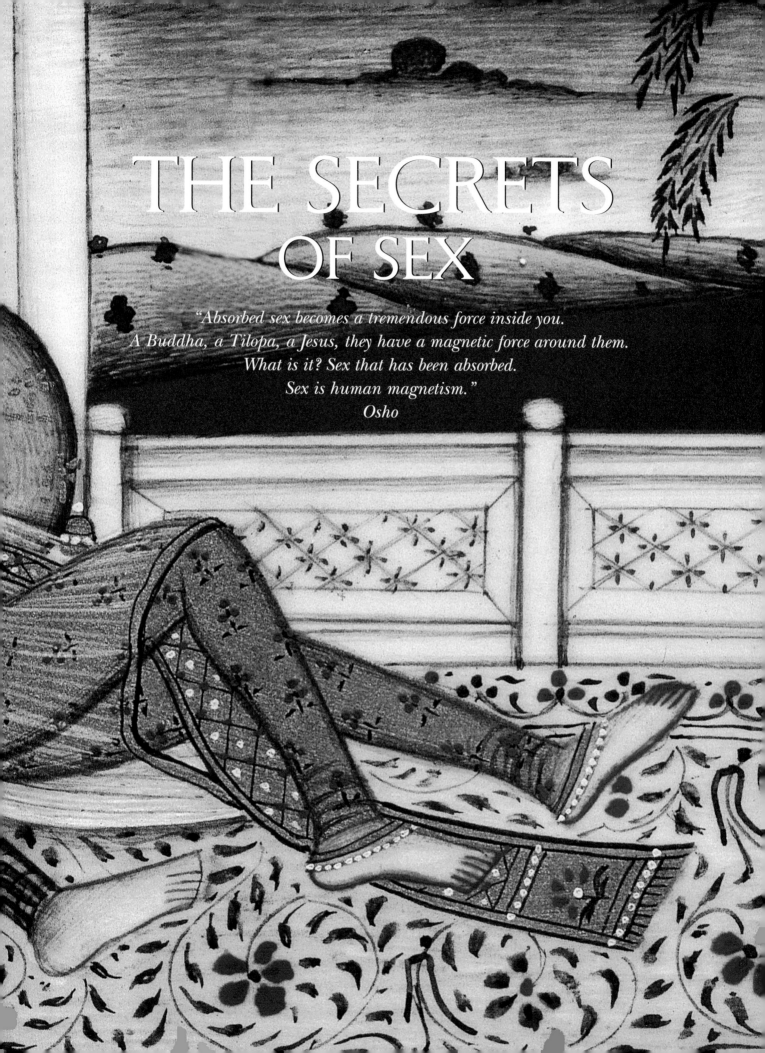

THE SECRETS
OF SEX

*"Absorbed sex becomes a tremendous force inside you.
A Buddha, a Tilopa, a Jesus, they have a magnetic force around them.
What is it? Sex that has been absorbed.
Sex is human magnetism."*
Osho

PATH
to Unity

In our society, sex has been considered sinful,
when in reality it is a natural act free of connotations.
With Tantra, it becomes a way to achieve unity and
higher levels of consciousness.

I like to know the etymology of words because we often use them without really knowing their meaning. The word "sex" is curious: it is derived from "sectus," which means "to cut" or "to divide," and certainly sex is something that has divided humanity, as much as football, politics, or religion. There are count-less examples of attempts to separate men and women, from schools that are all girls or all boys, to bunks in ships that are only for men or women. All because we discount the energetic law that says the more separated lo-vers are, the more attraction they feel. Romeo and Juliet, for example, can't consummate their love, and the desi-re only burns stronger. The more you deny something, the greater the urge to have it; the more you repress sex, the more you think about it.

In Tantra, on the other hand, sex is a means to a spiritual end of unity, which we must think about without losing sight of polarities. You will see feminine and masculine intermixing in everything around you, mutually ba-lancing each other.

Sex continues to be a secret for the majority of humanity because they lack understanding because they ha-ven't talked about or learned about it. Sex offers two beings the marvelous possibility to feel like one conscious-ness, melting away moral and social barriers.

A NEW LOOK AT ADAM AND EVE

There is a myth that has been misunderstood, and I ask divine inspiration to help me explain it: We have been told that there existed Adam and Eve, the serpent, the apple, and the tree of knowledge of good and evil. Now, if we see it from a tantric perspective, we discover that when God said, "This fruit you shall not eat," he didn't refer to the apple but rather to ejaculation. Why? Because if a man does not waste this energy, the fruit of energetic practice transforms into spiritual power, allowing a direct connection to God from the seventh chakra.

When a man ejaculates, energy drops from the seventh chakra (spiritual) to the first (material), and he experiences a feeling of separation, loneliness, and loss. The word "sin" means "to miss the mark," and this "error" was to eat (waste) the forbidden fruit instead of making it ascend the spine.

And what about the rest of the symbolism? The tree of knowledge is the vertebral column of man; the apple is red like the first chakra; and the serpent is kundalini as it is represented in the East. It is well known that he who seeks to awaken this energy and make it climb the backbone like a cobra to the highest chakra (site of spiritual communication) will discover that we are one with God!

There's one more thing: if we take the last "a" out of "Adan" (Adam in Spanish), we discover that the name is the same as "ADN" (DNA in Spanish): the genetic code of humanity.

I want to clarify that the meaning I have given these important symbols is from a personal lens and does not come from any tradition.

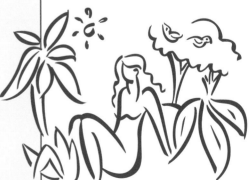

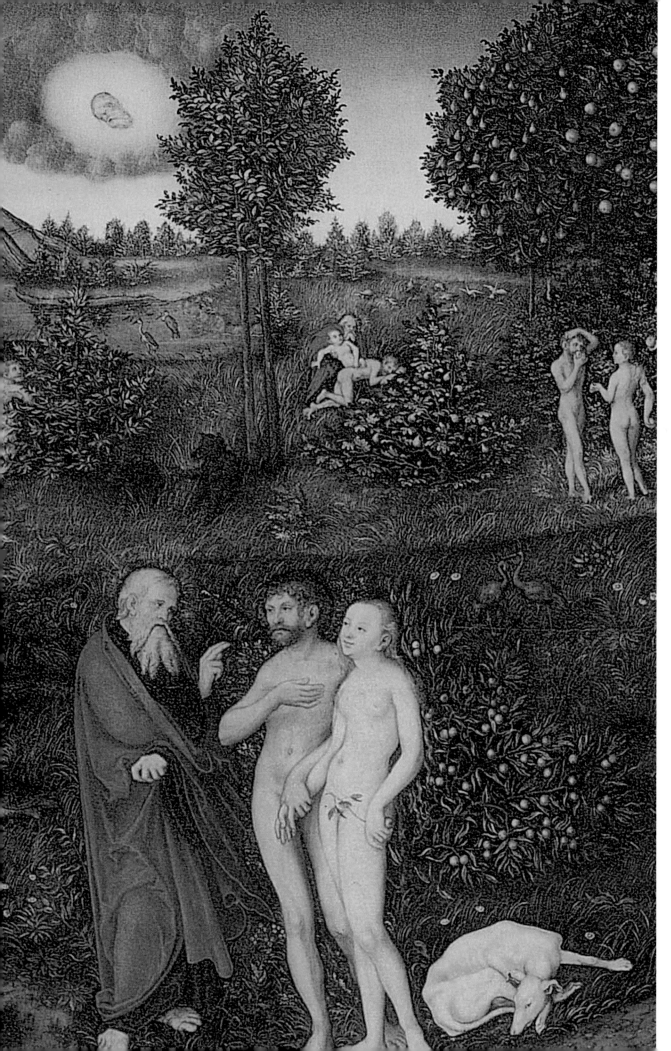

The biblical myth of Adam and Eve, and their expulsion from paradise, can be explained from a tantric perspective that gives the symbols surprising meanings.

THE MYSTERY OF DESIRE

Desire is the cause of existence and the whole world is moved by it. It's no coincidence that our planet is called "Kama Loka," "world of desires." If you fulfill a desire, you get satisfaction and happiness, while if you don't, you are depressed.

Desire should not be denied, but rather completed and transcended because it is in our nature to be dissatisfied. You want to eat at noon and when you finish you're already thinking about dinner.

Think about yourself for a moment. What do you desire? Where does your energy go each day? What would happen if your desire comes true?

You work because you want to express yourself and earn money; you seek sex with a partner because you desire their body and to share energy; you want to eat good food; you want to love and be loved; you want to be creative; you want to have power

and knowledge; you want a spiritual world and connection with divinity. Everyone seeks satisfaction from their desires, and until you are enlightened, this is the language you understand. Even the desire to have no desires is, itself, a desire.

You have to understand that we possess seven basic desires, which are directly related to each chakra and are the basis of the human experience. Tantra seeks to satisfy and balance these desires so we don't repress or deny any.

It's important to know what you desire. In fact, the art we need to learn is to manage our desires, identify our center so we don't lose it or identify with a desire. If you seek money and your mind is always thinking about it, this is logical because an important part (the base) is not realized. But this is just one aspect of life and we should learn not to identify with it so much. One wish is just that, and the consciousness shouldn't get stuck on it. The task is

to unstick and depersonalize; understand that you are a human being and naturally need to satisfy desires, but without putting too much stake in it. It's not that you need to move to the Himalayas to avoid desire: that would be unnatural. Those who do, do it out of fear or previous failure. It's very positive to do an inner cleanse at times in order to advance on your spiritual path, but only to strengthen you to later return to the world.

Know what you want, choose which desires will make you grow, and look for a path guided by your divinity to attain them. We all have the keys to realize our dreams and soul's desires.

FEMALE ORGASM AND EJACULATION

It's hard to believe that many women have never experienced an orgasm.

The beautiful word "orgasm" comes from the same root as "organism," "organization" or "organ." My definition of orgasm is "explosion of light in the cells."

Particularly in women (since they are sexually much stronger than men), the orgasm is a bridge of spiritual connection, a sacred instant where there is no mind, moral, thought, fear, or repression. Connected to ecstasy, Shakti awakens her kundalini, which runs from sacrum to head, bathing her in light and banishing physical and psychological limits.

A woman who experiences an orgasm is no longer the same. It will surprise you to know that the tongue is connected to the sexual center, the genitals. That's why when you kiss someone with your tongue, sexual energy is automatically awakened. Remember, on the other hand, a woman who talks a lot or gossips is not developing or satisfying her sexual energy.

For women, orgasms are the door that connects them to the divine. Since women carry their energy more

52

THE ANDROGYNE

For Tantra, the first origin was the androgyne; a being that was half masculine and half feminine later separated into man and woman. In fact, even today every human being is divided in two halves, since the left side of the body is feminine and the right is masculine.

The game (since life is a game of learning) consists in finding your Shiva or your Shakti once more, your sacred part, your other body to share mutually. But until this happens, you find other halves that aren't yours that you share moments with, learning, for some time, through multiple experiences. The goal

of all this is your evolution. But careful! You are already complete; you already have light, and only when you discover what you are, what you have, what you can share, can you give what you have. And although you can also be fine alone, the tantric proverb says **"A Shiva without his Shakti is a shava,"** meaning that a man without a woman is a corpse, and vice versa.

Relationships between partners, however, have become a serious subject and they suffer for lack of play. We've lost the ability to have fun and we've become rigid, fearful, and less spontaneous. Life loses joy if we don't play. Find your androgyne!

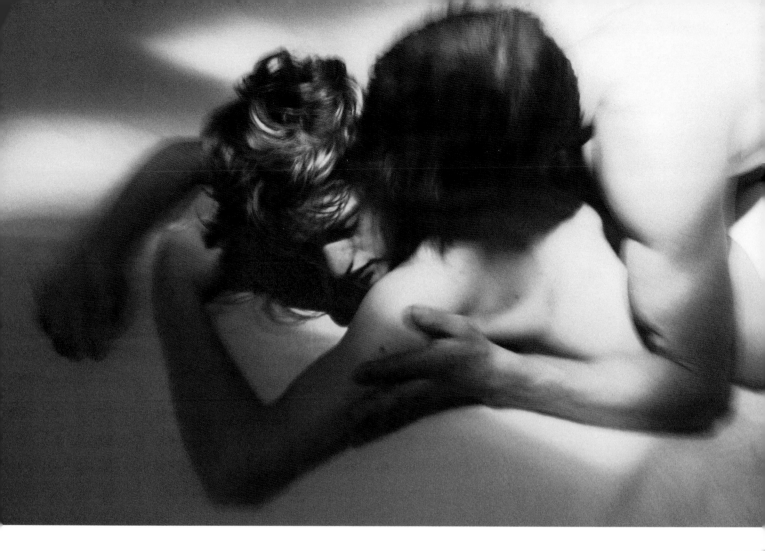

toward the interior (they implode) it is much easier for them to reach their inner world. Men, on the other hand, have their genitals on the outside and detonate outwardly (they explode), so it is much more difficult for them to reach their inner world.

But women can also ejaculate; it's called *amrita* and it is a white sticky liquid with highly energetic properties.

A woman, when she awakens her inner Shakti, can have multiple orgasms in a single sex act, giving her an inner state of happiness and fulfillment. Many women don't know the latent potential they have and end up deprived of this great experience.

What exactly does a Shakti's orgasm feel like? It's similar to a tickle, to feeling the body filled with electricity; it's an electrifying sensation that can't be controlled. The whole body is desire in

When a woman awakens her inner Shakti, she can achieve multiple orgasms, giving her a state of inner bliss.

the moment of orgasm; it is complete, like a spiritual drug. All of her skin is stimulated and the sensation of time, space, and mind disappear completely.

As for differences, a clitoral orgasm is stronger than one from G-spot stimulation. The basic differences are the contractions; in the clitoral or-

gasm there are seven or eight strong contractions in succession, at times even three to five orgasms in a row. The G-spot orgasm feels similar but without contractions.

Many women can relate to this description; others don't know what it's like. Tantra has a higher rung that allows women to take off to brighter skies, to ascend the discharge of energy up the spine, igniting the chakras to the top and fusing with the divinity they possess. It provides the potential to eliminate the ego and enlarge the soul.

The orgasm is a spiritual experience available to humans, since it connects to a state of bliss, eroticism, devotion, love, depersonalization, and spiritual universality, and gives the sensation of a return to the cosmic home. With an orgasm, the divine hand rests on the individual soul.

FOR HIM: ORGASM WITHOUT EJACULATION

Men are too "primitive" in their sexual relationships, but luckily Tantra is gaining popularity. With its popularity comes a less yang form of sexuality that helps men understand women more, as women have most often suffered abuse from men.

Modern man lives with too much haste: he competes, he stresses about his schedule, he tries to earn money and prestige (or just make it to the end of the month), etc. When he is with a woman, he ejaculates quickly.

For Tantra, it is vital not to ejaculate (or at least do it only every ten to fifteen sex acts) in order to conserve energy (bindu) to use creatively in other facets of life.

The mind, breathing, and ejaculation are connected. When you breathe quickly and unevenly, without rhythm, ejaculation is imminent; desire disappears and the penis (lingam) falls as if into an abyss.

Getting back in the mood requires time for rest, food, and new accumulation of desire.

> **Mind, breathing, and ejaculation are connected. When a man breathes rapidly and unevenly, ejaculation is imminent.**

Tantra provides excellent techniques to prevent ejaculation (detailed in the practice section of the book). When there is no ejaculation, you can elevate energy with inner consciousness, to transform the seminal explosion to orgasmic implosion: an electric current that goes from the sacrum to the brain. It produces a bioenergetic alchemy and transforms carnal sex to a spiritual experience. The masculine orgasm is a discharge of energetic magnetism that every man has inside and can be called Shiva, the dancing divinity in the form of a man.

Life is dance for Tantra, and in this moment the common, mortal man can incarnate divine grandeur and feel the great touch of infinity. Mind, ego, and machismo are dead; the doors to transcendence are open.

Any man that uses a little intelligence can open himself to Tantra and its teachings. The old era of machismo is done. Women are coming with force for equal rights, as much sexual as social.

When you begin to investigate yourself, to experiment with sensations, your psyche and emotions change for the better. Ejaculation is no longer necessary; one can prolong the sexual act for hours, and desire does not end but even grows greater. And the woman will benefit as much as the man. Men look for other women when their desire runs out, and desire runs out from excessive ejaculation, among other reaons.

54

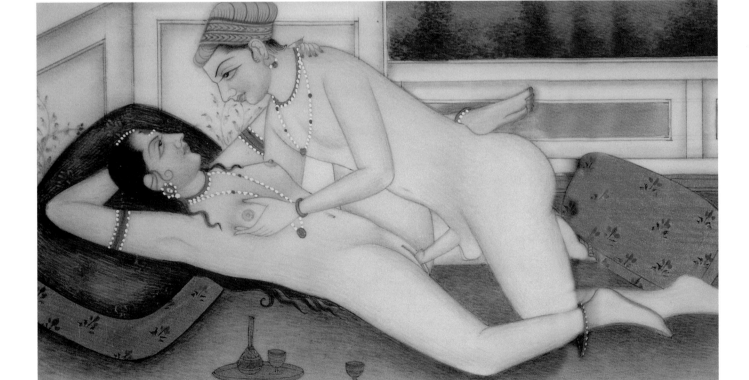

What's more, prostate problems have a lot to do with this; semen, like blood, can't be produced scientifically, it is magic and irreplaceable. Remember that man and woman generate electricity and magnetism, and this is what unites them. The attraction is energetic. Careful! A wise man prevents problems. Don't waste your desire, don't waste your bindu!

When you learn the techniques for not ejaculating, in order to transform this sacred energy, all of your talents (love, intelligence, inner power, and creativity) will awaken like a forest in the morning, full of fragrance and sound.

WHAT TO DO WITH THE ENERGY

The transmutation, guide, and focus of energy is vitally important, because when man and woman awaken their kundalini they must control it.

It is an energetic law that energy responds to your thoughts. After two or three hours of tantric sex, the energy fields are very strong, luminous, and magnetic; they absorb prana from the bodies and the environment. The energy has developed and now you must do something with it. I recommend meditating, dancing, painting, singing, writing, decorating, generating new ideas or plans, cooking, woodworking, or any other creative activity. The tremendous impulse after tantric sex will take you to a state of total bliss, peace, and inner depth. Use this energy creatively.

It's important to keep in mind when you practice tantric sex and awaken so much energy, if you don't channel it, it will take its own path. For example, it might alter the liver, producing anger or disputes. You may become irritable from not focusing it in a creative channel. Since sexual energy is fire, it will burn wood (liver).

After the ritual, you and your partner should take time to practice meditation to channel energy. There's no need to make love in a hurry; Tantra doesn't heed the clock. You

OJAS SHAKTI

SEXUAL ENERGY TRANSFORMED INTO SPIRITUAL ENERGY
Tantric transmutation is called "Ojas Shakti," which means "spiritual oil."

It's not that semen experiences a transformation, but rather that it is the raw material. The process nourishes the spiritual potency of a person, centers them, and enriches the consciousness. This sacred oil rises along the astral column, through the central channel sushamna, strengthening the chakras and awakening the talents they possess. Its greatest merit is the expansion of the consciousness and the internal cleansing it produces. Each person is a world and harbors diverse feelings, repressed emotions, conflicts, and fears. Tantric purification is strong; often times painful and unexplainable. Immersing ourselves in knowledge of our spiritual life offers us many rooms: dark and empty as often as luminous, or full of past pains. You must be brave, conscious, and intelligent to allow cleansing. Sexual energy transformed into spiritual energy will give you the key to open all your inner rooms. And with *practice and consciousness, the energy will naturally take the enlightened path where it belongs.*

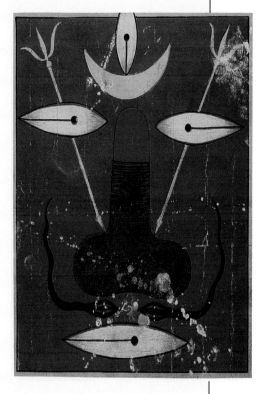

should take consciousness that you are on the path to becoming an artist of love and sex, and every artist needs time to complete their work.

"BIG BANG": THE COSMIC ORGASM?

The Bible says that "in the beginning was the Word": the Orientals talk about the OM (the original sound); and scientists assert that the Big Bang was the great explosion that initiated creation.

Tantra bases its cosmic genesis on the principle of unity: the One not manifested that is revealed through the creation of the two sacred polarities, Shiva (the masculine) and Shakti (the feminine), the balance and harmony that today continue to create numberless forms. Creation begins from the One via masculine and feminine

energy, which, when "put in motion," generates a sound, an infinite explosion of luck and energy, of perfection in motion. If what we call God, Tao, One, or Absolute is perfect, this perfection and energy of happiness have exploded into millions upon millions of different forms, lives, and galaxies: many more than the human mind can comprehend.

With the infinite zone of my being, I like to think or intuit that the One was so complete, so full of pleasure, that it expanded in a cosmic orgasm, and that the creation of life on this and other planets and galaxies is the orgasm of God, a super powered stage of eternal delight freely distributing itself to infinity.

FEAR OF SEX

Wrong ideas about sin, guilt, fear, punishment, and good and evil have destroyed the natural and spontaneous nature of human beings. We have been erroneously taught that if desire emerges, it must be repressed, and the consequence as been all sorts of fantasies, depravations, and derivations of sexual energy. If desire comes, what is wrong with loving and being one being for a moment? Why burden sex with a "moral" connotation? Why are scenes of violence and death in movies not condemned when scenes of lovemaking are censured? Have you ever stopped to think that they've pulled the wool over your eyes, that you've handed in your freedom to others? Death, bombs, and catastrophes are common currency in the news, but sexual scenes or someone sunbathing nude on

> Sex is a natural phenomenon, something so sacred it cannot be a product of fear.

the beach cause a big stir. The body and sex have been so repressed that seeing it has become surprising. Energy awakens in every moment and you can't deny it.

The way of controlling people, of taking their freedom and making them dependent on religions or the powerful has been done through repression and fear. If you adopt a tantric point of view, you will see two energies that respond to the call of nature and follow the path of attraction. What is it that

attracts them deep down? It's not just the physical form or beauty, but the energy they give off. And if you deeply desire the body, the delight, you will also want the sensation of unity, of knowing you are not alone.

Sex is a natural phenomenon. You are born, united, and shared through sex. And something so sacred cannot be a product of fear, but only a natural understanding. It is profane to use sex as an outlet, to use another as an object, something that Tantra rejects because it is a loss of vitality.

Immerse yourself without fear in sex; you will learn more about yourself and the hidden ability to understand the paths that have generated life.

SEXUAL REPRESSION

For a long time, woman has been censored; society has prohibited the movement of her hips, covered her in veils, condemned and defaced her. Pale, she has lost the light in her eyes, and the power of Shakti has been buried. Obviously, so much repression has made many women submissive.

Today, however, women have once again awakened the feminine power. They take care of themselves, they have economic autonomy, they invest in beauty. All good tantric qualities, but they still haven't shed the years of Catholicism and sexist education, which has given them emotional armor, unnatural ideas, and repressed energies that characterize the body.

With physical force, man has imposed his "laws." It's amazing how a husband can condemn the free erotic spirit of his wife, making her a languid housewife, and then go to the prostitute around the corner in search of pleasure. What a hypocrite! Women have been repressed so much they have even been forced to take the last name of the husband, as if she were an object. To be fair, the man should also add the woman's last name to his own.

THE CROWN JEWEL

The clitoris is an organ of the female body whose sole function is to give pleasure. Curiously, nature has created a zone that awakens eroticism and bioenergy, and lights the sexual fire. It is a small point at the door of the yoni that fills every centimeter of skin with effervescence. Tantra calls it "the crown jewel" and it is respected, stimulated, and worshiped with the fingers and tongue, unlike other cultures that practice abhorrent female circumcision. Why should man take away what God has created? The tantric vision is that everything on Earth should be used, or if it's not used, at least let it be.

Tantra stimulates the clitoris so that energy travels like electricity through the bodies and initiates the feedback, the nourishment of vital energy, the tantric circle.

A woman can stimulate her clitoris without a partner, with her fingers, and use circular breathing techniques to awaken her energy. The body is sacred and should be explored and experienced. "He who knows the reality of the body, knows the reality of the universe," says a tantric proverb.

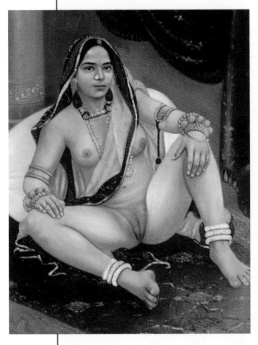

56

Repression generates more desire; a person who represses sex will think about it constantly, in how to avoid it, but the energy goes where thought does, growing like a snowball. The basic cause of sexual repression is power: the woman, with the movement of her hips, a simple glance, or the toss of her sensual hair, can bring down an entire empire (Cleopatra drove men crazy with just her perfume). Men fear sharing power, so they have repressed women.

It's very easy for a man to lose his consciousness when he falls in love; for this he has possessed rather than loved freely. Tantra proposes intelligent love, consciousness balanced with energy, but it's a skill you have to develop, a work of art to sculpt. You are yourself evolving.

Remember that what you repress will be what you later emphasize most. It will be there, hidden, crouching, waiting to come out. Women have all sorts of fantasies because of dissatisfaction and repression, but now the feminine energy has awoken all around the planet and is trying to free itself and take its natural place. Just look at all the magazine covers; almost all of them are women, free and beautiful. The universal consciousness is trying to free the Shakti and bless this wounded planet with her virtues.

PSYCHIC PROTECTION

Training in Tantra includes an aspect related to psychic and energetic protection.

Many people have felt heaviness, yawning, and gloom entering a busy place or in a meeting with lots of people. There are techniques to avoid losing energy in these instances, or during sex, that you can practice alone or with a partner before maithuna.

Energy can be lost through the nine orifices in the body—the mouth, the nose, the two ears, two eyes, the top of the head, the anus, the

THE G-SPOT

Both women and men have a pleasure point in their genitals connected with the brain called the "G-spot." It was discovered in the Western world thanks to Ernest Grafberger, a scientist who discovered it in the upper part of the vagina (yoni), a cavity full of nerve endings directly connected to the area of the brain that produces pleasure hormones. This zone, easily stimulated with a finger, is the size of a small nut, and its only function is to give pleasure. Tantrics have known about it for millennium and use it to awaken the kundalini. Men also have a G-spot: it's located in the anus, and its upper cavity is also full of nerve endings similar to those found in the female body. This spot can be stimulated in Shiva as much as Shakti, allowing the yin energy that everyone has to manifest.

The waves of pleasure and energy that run through the cells, meridians, and the skin awaken endless new emotions and sensations for many; however, it shouldn't be over stimulated because the opposite can occur, producing discomfort. It is a detonator to raise bioenergy that the consciousness will channel tantrically through the central channel and the chakras.

In anal sex, the woman can have powerful orgasms through G-spot stimulation, due to the strong tremors and energetic waves that kundalini provokes. If this happens to you, don't

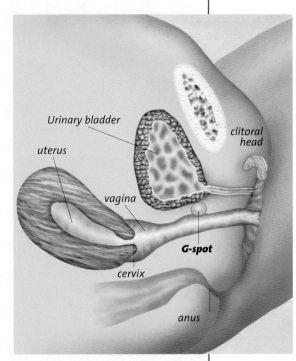

be afraid; it is the breaking down of repression and the manifestation of the sacred in your body. Breathing and inner consciousness can be helpful in this moment to let yourself go freely from the sacrum to the top of the head.

lingam or yoni—but also through the fingertips, toes, pores, navel, and especially through the energetic body. The technique consists of visualizing these orifices while closing them with the middle and index fingers. This ritual of psychic protection, known as nyasa, can be accompanied by the mantra OM and visualization of the cosmic egg (the body of one or both lovers enclosed in a blue circle).

Mahanirvana Tantra recommends beginning by touching the top of the head, then continuing through the forehead, eyes, ears, earlobes, nostrils, cheeks, lips, teeth, chin, neck, fingerips, palms, wrists, arms, forearms, shoulders, chest, heard, stomach, thighs, knees, insteps, toes, and finally, sex organ.

Take the fingertips across each indicated point while maintaining a strong inner state and visualize a seal in each point. It can also be done with kisses instead of fingers. Nyasa strengthens erotic energy at the same time as reducing loss of energy. Remember that all magical traditions have protection techniques. Use them to prevent harmful energy from interfering with your magic act.

SIDDHIS

The completion of ancient sexual rituals, as well as those that couples do today, will awaken innate natural capacities in the human being. Siddhis, or extrasensory powers, are not a goal in and of themselves, but the result of practice on the path to a state of Samadhi.

Tantra tells us that siddhis can be obtained through meditation, sex without orgasm, pranayamas, mantras, fasting, and contact with fire. One who has obtained paranormal powers and risen above the limitations of the physical plane is called Siddha Yogi.

The powers range from an extreme sexual capacity to intuition, clairvoyance, telepathy, and a connection with the higher spiritual world.

BRAHMACHARYA

The state of Brahmacharya has been misunderstood as meaning "absence of sexual activity," when really it means completing the sex act without spilling semen. "Brahmacharya" means "Master Brahma" (one has become Brahma) and it is a state that gives a man great potency, having transmuted his seminal energy into spiritual energy. Sex becomes a magical and alchemic act, nourishing itself with energy and generating the combustion necessary so that the kundalini rises, rather than sinking through semen and losing the fruit of sadhana.

Celibacy is unnatural and harmful to mental health. A person that doesn't have sex for a long time runs the risk of losing their mental capacities if they don't transmute this energy into art, service, or fraternal love. Tantra recommends making love regularly without losing energy. You can ejaculate once a month during the full moon, offering the energy to the cosmic Shakti, or a particular wish you want to come true.

Brahmacharya is the man capable of having sexual activity without losing his bindu, storing his energy to develop his spiritual destiny.

SEXUAL INITIATION

The first initiation of every living being is through the yoni of the mother, given that birth represents the entrance into the current life and the forgetting of previous lives. The other initiations come from taking consciousness during sex, although there are also advanced initiations in dreams. In every act of tantric sexual initiation, there is a flow of energy, a stimulus of the senses, and an awakening of transcendental consciousness. In tantric tradition, the woman is the initiator. In ancient times, the woman embodied the role of guru and initiated partners, especially at midnight during the fifteen days of dark moon or during eclipses. Initiations are meant to awaken the sacred secrets of sex: the strengthening of positive experiences; bringing energy to the chakras; waking the kundalini; and entering a state of supraconsciousness. There are various tantric rituals of initiation:

1.Chakra Puja

It means "circular worship," and energy is channeled and exchanged consciously between partners (usually eight) that make up the circle. It consists of stopping before reaching orgasm so that the next partner begins to heighten the eros, and so on. In this way, they create an incredibly powerful accumulation of energy, creating a vortex that charges the chakras of all the participants. The ritual imparts spiritual ecstasy on all of the participants, awakening their mystic inner abilities.

2. Bhairavi Chakra

It is a ritual to the goddess Kali. Form a circle of three, five, seven, or nine participants in sexual activity. When there are nine, it represents the energies of the nine planets and liberates the karma of the participants. This ritual begins and ends with paying homage to the feminine principle. You can worship this principle with a small statute, an object of devotion, fruit, and incense, or just by taking consciousness of the inner Shakti. These rituals are not an excuse for a wild orgy, but a form of strengthening spiritual power in all of the chakras and elevating the consciousness and kundalini.

3.Yogini Chakra

This is practiced between a man and three, five, seven, or nine women. The man and his partner sit in the middle surrounded by a circle of eight yoginis that intervene in the sexual game. This liberates and circulates the yin energy to the maximum. Each of the eight women gives herself to the man and he must not spill his bindu (semen) on any of them. The man absorbs the energy of the eight women and then provides his seed, full of power, to the ninth, his partner. In ancient times this ritual was practiced by emperors, kings, or tantrics to conceive children.

58

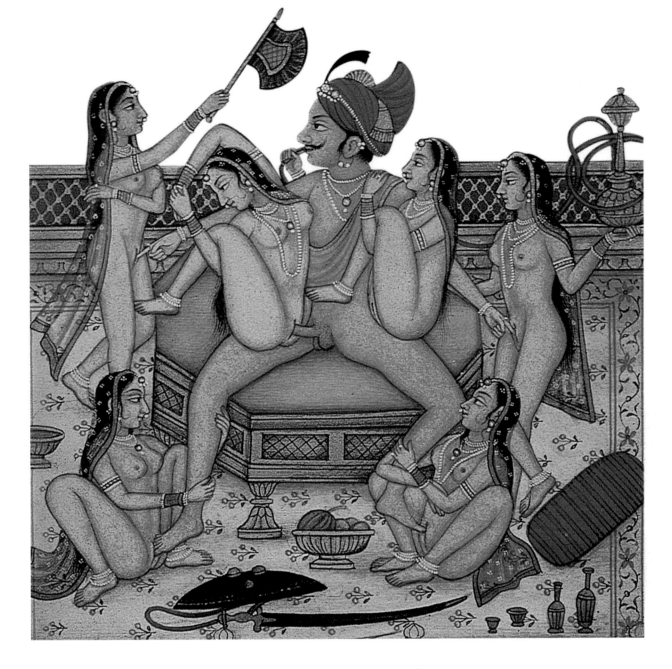

EROTIC FANTASIES

Tantra has some visualizations of erotic fantasies that provoke energy to awaken and circulate. The Prapanchasara Tantra says: "Think of a beautiful garden full of trees that grant wishes and fragrant flowers, in harmony with the rhythmic buzzing of great bees. Then meditate on Vishnu, seated on the great bird Garuda, which rests on a red lotus. This form of Vishnu is red, expressing erotic feeling, splendid as a hibiscus flower and shining with the force of millions of new suns. Vishnu manifests as a handsome young man who emanates sweet nectar and loving

Sex becomes a magical act in which energy ascends rather than being lost.

goodness. He holds various weapons, including a conch shell, a club, a bow, and a discus, and his eyes are fixed on the face of his partner Lakshmi, who embraces him with all of her love. Around this divine couple are many beautiful women with big

thighs, hips, and breasts, who smile erotically, moving voluptuously and imitating with their hands the sensual shape of the lotus. Their lips are open but they are silent, in a type of tremulous passion. With their clothes and hair in disarray, they clearly express their eroticism."

When a person fantasizes, it generates desire and automatically awakens energy. Fantasies can be used at the beginning of the act, as a type of meditation, and can be about anything, but once the energy is moving you must center yourself in what's real, in the cosmic partner, and share them both in the present moment.

COUPLES AND THIRDS

Hindu texts affirm that you can heighten emotions with the presence of a third (Bharata), and the *Kama Sutra* says: "When a man makes love to two women he loves equally, it is called 'United Position.'" Although Tantra emphasizes the divine couple, it doesn't oppose anything that helps the soul grow.

The sex act can occur between two women and a man because women are naturally receptive and between most of them is a feeling of sisterhood, sensuality, and eroticism that generates attraction and unity.

A multiple encounter is called "Secret Game" and it was done by emperors, kings, and divinities in all cultures. Muhommad had nine wives; Krishna had an entourage of 108 gopis that adored him; in some African tribes, women formed partnerships and then found a man; and oriental emperors practiced magic sex with multiple women—obviously without losing energy, accumulating powerful yin energy with which to rule and obtain paranormal powers.

> **Tantra accepts sex between three or more participants if it is done for spiritual ends.**

The *Chandamaharosana Tantra* mentions: "A woman of the moon is enjoyed by someone similar. The third person differs from the other two and balances their forces. By taking pleasure together, they are all freed from decadence and death. The right and the left combine in the central path. He stimulates both of them; they excite each other mutually and combine with him. The two moons are always full of nectar and the sun burns but doesn't burn out."

There is a Western stereotype that monogamy causes divorce and conflict, as well as infidelity and cheating. For Tantra, sex between three or more participants is acceptable only if it is for spiritual ends, for the accumulation of energy in the chakras and rituals of power.

Maharajas and kings, as well as those initiated in the metaphysical secrets of sex, have used the "ritual of the five senses," that is, the union of a man with five women, each representing a different sense. In this way, the five senses were stimulated to obtain spiritual liberation, Samadhi, although it can also be used as a fantasy without doing it for real. For example, once a couple has raised each of their kundalinis to the highest chakra, they should visualize a beautiful red Dakini, full of magical powers, with whom they will identify to obtain wisdom and realization of dreams. This is practicing the sexual magic of Tantra.

When a Union of Three occurs, the energies must be channeled through breathing, visualization, the extension of pleasure, the opening of the chakras, and control of the orgasm. The sexual points of the body—sex organs, mouths, breasts, hands, and feet—should be stimulated, and the loss of energy through the navel or crown should be avoided. The consciousness is put in the wave of connection between the human and the divine, in a state of total acceptance and submission. In order for the Union of Three to occur naturally, it should not consider personality, personal interests, or strong emotions, since this would make it mundane and farther from the tantric goal of spiritual liberation and transcendence. Both Shaktis must embody the feminine power, giving themselves to the man with total devotion and joy as if he were the incarnation of Shiva himself.

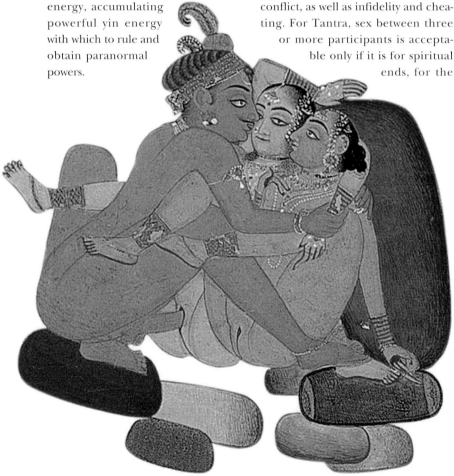

THOUGHT, RESPIRATION, AND EJACULATION

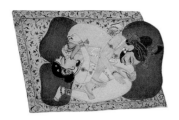

ORAL SEX

It's amazing how many people smoke. Without realizing the hidden meaning of this bad habit, they continue lighting up over and over again. It has to do with an oral fixation caused by deprivations suffered during childhood. When a baby is born, the first thing they do is cut the umbilical cord. This is an abrupt act followed by bright lights that blind the newborn. The baby has gone nine months in darkness and dependent on the umbilical cord, and now it must breathe or die; there is no other alternative and it is highly stressful for the infant. On top of that, months later it will nurse from the mother's breast and if the period of breastfeeding is insufficient, as an adult the individual will miss this state when there were no worries and will seek out toxic cigarettes to replace the breast milk and amniotic fluid. He will also talk a lot, a product of not having satisfied the oral phase. Frequently, a baby will suck its fingers, even inside the womb before being born, and this means that every human being should be respected as an individual; also, later he will look for substitutes for the maternal archetype.

What is the tantric therapy for quitting smoking? Oral sex is a (always pleasurable) way to change a harmful habit for a constructive one. For women as well as men, it will satiate oral craving, but if you are traditional or have moral objections to doing it, you can try taking a bottle of juice, milk, or some drink (avoid alcohol) to bed at night, so you can also have the same effect.

It may surprise you to know that the majority of my students did not have a long period of breast-feeding. Although Tantra teaches through play and laugh-

One of the greatest metaphysical secrets of sex revealed by Tantra is that ejaculation is directly related to respiration and thought. Sexual excitation provokes agitated breathing, and an agitated mind causes premature ejaculation. If a tantric yogi governs his breathing, he also governs his mind, and can delay or even prevent ejaculation. Through diverse breathing techniques, you can achieve a high level of energy and make it circulate through energetic channels. The protection of mantras and visualization of mandalas stabilizes the mind. An important oriental text says: "In love making, semen should be considered an extremely precious substance." In saving it, the man protects his life. After every ejaculation, the loss of semen is recuperated by absorbing essential liquids from the woman. There is a method of saving semen that consists of a nine beats after every nine penetrations. The emission of semen is also avoided by pressing a point located below the lingam with the fingers of the left hand. This technique helps prevent external emission, making it return to the body and thus strengthening the whole body. To absorb the essence of the woman, alternate nine light thrusts with one deep penetration. Aligning your mouth with your partner's, inhale their breath and drink their saliva. Once swallowed, this descends to the stomach and the yin essence is transformed into yang essence. Do this three time, then give light thrusts, interspersing one deep one for each nine shallow ones, until you've complete nine series of nine thrusts. This number, eighty-one, signifies the complete realization of yang.

As we see, sex is not something unimportant or to be done in a hurry. For Tantra, it is a science and an art that contains metaphysical transcendental secrets. The retention of energetic seed is vital for spiritual transformation. Kalachakra Tantra maintains: "Respiration, thought, and semen are the three elements of potential for enlightenment." They should be harmonized and consciously controlled. The yogi that unites respiration, thought, and semen becomes the Indestructable, gifted with transcendental spontaneity. This is an invaluable secret to life and tantric sex. Learn it, meditate on it, and practice it; it is a personal journey from animal impulse to divine desire.

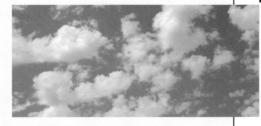

ter, do not think that this is a joke. Do a test and experiment before you deny it. Tantra considers the sex organs sacred, not just sources of pleasure: the yoni is worshiped as the door to life from which we have all come, while the lingam is taken by women as a phallic symbol of the power that generates life.

SEXUAL ALCHEMY

Learning to transmute sexual energy will give your life a big push.

Tantra tries to alchemize the material, spiritualize it, and sex is the first step (and the most physical). Alchemy will reveal the essence of life. Sex is like the grapes and the spiritual result of tantric alchemy is wine.

This wine will allow you to enjoy the pleasures of the body and the talents of the soul. You can make good meals, have meditative sex, dance, sing, and be with your partner under the Moon and the stars. For once, turn off the TV! Tantra will make you a Dionysus, a sensitive being, fun, deep, with consciousness, movement, and enthusiasm, full of vitality. Just as Dionysus was the Greek god of wine, celebration, and pleasure (he traveled and celebrated with a caravan accompanying him), now you can embody the Dionysian spirit of your life. A bit of fun, romance, adventure, depth, and mediation is the perfect formula for living in this world; a festive spirit that will come to the surface when, through tantric practices, you revive your inner talents that you possess.

Fun, romance, and meditation are the ingredients to the perfect formula for living in this world. Distance yourself from anything that doesn't give pleasure.

PLEASURE, JOY, AND CELEBRATION

If you had the chance to read *The Name of the Rose* by Umberto Eco, you will remember that the book was based on a macabre plan to keep people under control. It has to do with an order given by the Catholic Church banning a certain book, so they poison the edges of the pages. Whoever read it would certainly die. A very astute priest begins to investigate, and discovers the truth: the cursed book was banned because it was about . . . laughter!

Why would someone want you not to laugh? Because he who laughs is happy, and he who is happy is connected to God directly, without intermediaries. And who needs a "divine intermediary" if you can do it yourself? Why should a priest or a monk tell you what to do if you are already healthy and communicate with your own inner wisdom? How can you think that the divine is not in every part, outside and inside of you, in all the corners of the universe?

Pleasure, joy, laughter, and sex (sources of pleasure and transcendence) have been condemned, and psychological damage has been embedded deep in the human subconscious. Little by little, Tantra frees you from the conditioning that has filled your head. You can learn through pleasure, enjoyment, and being conscious; there is no need to be a saint or carry a weight that doesn't exist or belong to you. Responsibility is individual. There is no past guilt, and real life consists of living in the present with the five senses based in the present and personal experience.

Remember: Distance yourself from everything that doesn't give pleasure. God wants you to be happy and to enjoy life's lessons every day.

THE MORAL, THE GOOD, AND THE BAD

No matter how hard you look, there is no dividing line between good and evil, between moral and immoral. Just as it is moral for an Eskimo to lend his wife sexually to a foreigner, for a Westerner this is infidelity. Morality is subjective, as is the idea of good and evil. If a football fan asks God to let his team win the game this Sunday, it would be unjust for the other team. The problem lies in the fact that we only look outwardly, when what determines what is good or evil is internal, your conscience.

WITHOUT SEX THERE IS NO LIFE

A fundamental premise of Tantra is to consider everything sacred, without divisions or comparisons. Sex is sacred simply because it precedes the birth of a human being; because it is a moment in which you can share what you feel with your partner; and, in its deepest state, because it can regenerate you spiritually. The tantric eyes see sex as the first rung to ascend the sacred ladder to consciousness. Just as the more advanced a rocket is, the less equipment it needs, once you have awakened sexual energy you will deepen your inner states of spirituality and expanded consciousness. Have you ever stopped to think that without sex there would be no life on Earth? Without sex the continuity of the species would be in danger, since even plants have sex lives. Flowers contain the two polarities: the stem (yang, masculine) is a phallic symbol, and the open, receptive petals, the yoni full of life and fertility, is the principle, feminine yin. All of this should make us conscious that we need to recover the sacred respect for sex: think about it, live it, and experience it as a unique encounter of body and soul.

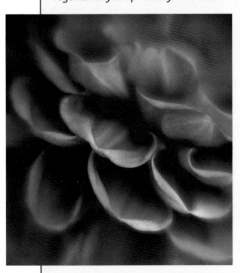

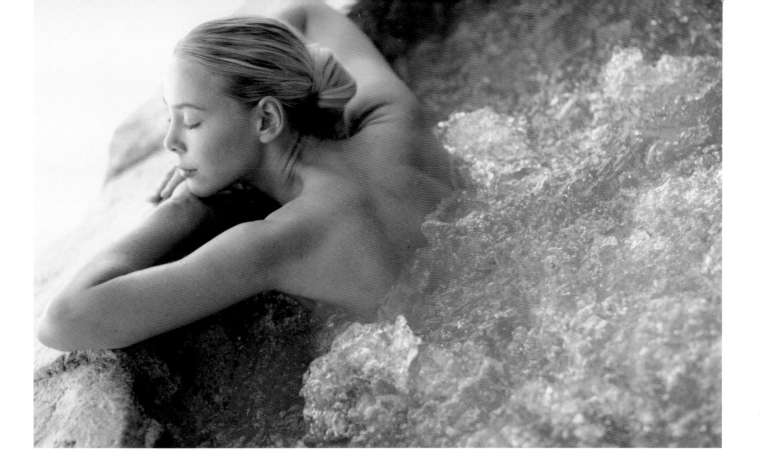

Tantra is not guided by notions of good or evil; rather, it believes in individual responsibility and consciousness. Are you aware, or are you asleep? Every mediation, experience, feeling, or song has to give you greater awareness in your life. You need to be more aware of the signs that the divine offers you.

As long as what you choose to do does not cause suffering to another, then it is okay to do, especially if it helps you grow in some manner. In any case, there is no guide or list of "moral and immoral acts." If it is productive, if it generates growth and awareness, then don't hesitate in doing it.

Finally, never allow anyone to dictate morality to you. Always use your own voice as a guide—the one connected to your heart—because this is the microphone that will allow you to communicate directly with the divine.

Because of ideas of morality, wars have been fought, magical people have been burnt, and many others have been decapitated. If you have read *The Scarlett Letter* by Nathaniel Hawthorne,

you will know that is about a repressed American society that hung the book's protagonist because she left a needle in a doll. The moral inquisitors meted out their justice because they accused her of practicing magic. They condemned an individual who was simply sowing, believing that she was purposefully sticking the doll with needles!

Human history includes a great amount of barbarity. It is time to soften the heart, give it wings, and to cease speculating and condemning. If someone guides themselves with their heart and their internal voice, everything that comes of it will simply be good.

COMMON SEX AND TANTRIC SEX

COMMON SEX	TANTRIC SEX
– Release of tension	– Regeneration of energy
– Rush to ejaculate	– By not ejaculating, you feel the global orgasm
– Ego remains	– Ego and duality disappear
– Division maintained	– Lovers fuse into the androgyne
– Energy lost	– Energy rises and energizes chakras
– Desire and passion spent	– Desire intensifies
– Climax reached, then a drop	– State of consciousness deepens
– Accelerates aging	– Elixir of longevity
– Personality remains	– Names are forgotten, union of souls achieved
– Fall into routine	– A magical ritual
– Limited to a short period of time	– Can last for hours

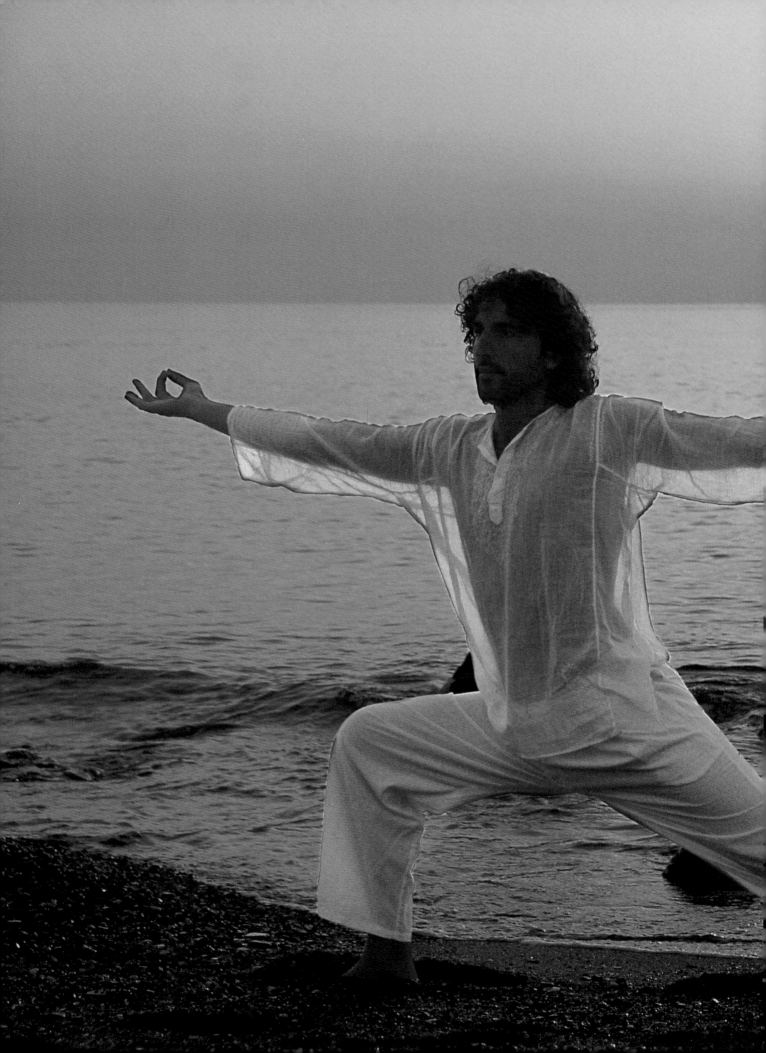

ENERGETIC
EXERCISES

*"Do your exercises with the tenacity and
zeal of an artist interested in producing a work of genius.
The work of genius is you, and the artist as well."*
Master Kuthumi

THE ELEVATION
of Energy

Each thought and movement carries the form of "prana,"
the cosmic force that maintains life.
Through yogic exercises called "pranayamas,"
we can capture this energy and nourish all the chakras.

Prana is the vital energy, the cosmic force that maintains life. It consists of negative ions, tiny packets of energy in its pure state, where all force resides: the force of attraction, of repulsion, gravity, electricity, etc. Without prana there is no life because the soul is all force and energy.

This primary principle is found everywhere: in the air, in food, in the water . . . But none of these are prana, only the simple vessel of it. The air—which is seventy-eight percent nitrogen, twenty-one percent oxygen, and the remainder other gases—is the theater where the great character, prana, plays the role of protagonist. It's brimming with free prana and the human being can most easily absorb it from fresh air through breathing. In normal respiration, we absorb some amount of prana; through tantric yoga breathing we can accumulate a greater reserve in the brain and the chakras to use when necessary.

Prana obeys the mind, thought, and visualization, although its command is thought, the key with which we can open or close the door of energy before us. Prana can be seen in the rays of the sun or in a clear sky over the sea, as if it were tiny sperm that move in the air.

Each activity, thought, and movement of the body carries the form of prana. The nervous force, for example, is a form of energy. Prana is linked with the most dynamic aspect of energy: the negative ions, high velocity particles of energy. On the other hand, positive ions are heavier. A shower can get rid of excess positive ions and reenergize us.

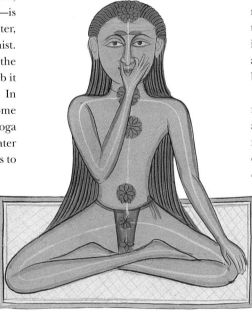

Material is energy in action; everything is in constant vibration at different frequencies, giving the impression of solid material. If we want to get to know prana more and learn to consciously accumulate more in our chakras, the first step is to govern the movement of the lungs, of breathing. Pranayama is the classic yoga breathing exercise to capture prana and nourish the chakras. It seeks to awaken another form of energy, the kundalini, the inner fire hidden in every human in the muladhara chakra.

To govern prana is to govern the mind, which can't operate without the help of prana, and which quiets if the breathing is also peaceful. As an ancient proverb says, "Learning to breathe is learning to live."

Turtles breathe four to six times per minute, and humans between fifteen and eighteen times. The turtle lives for a long time, so if we breathe softly, calmly, and slowly, it's likely that we can achieve longevity healthily and consciously.

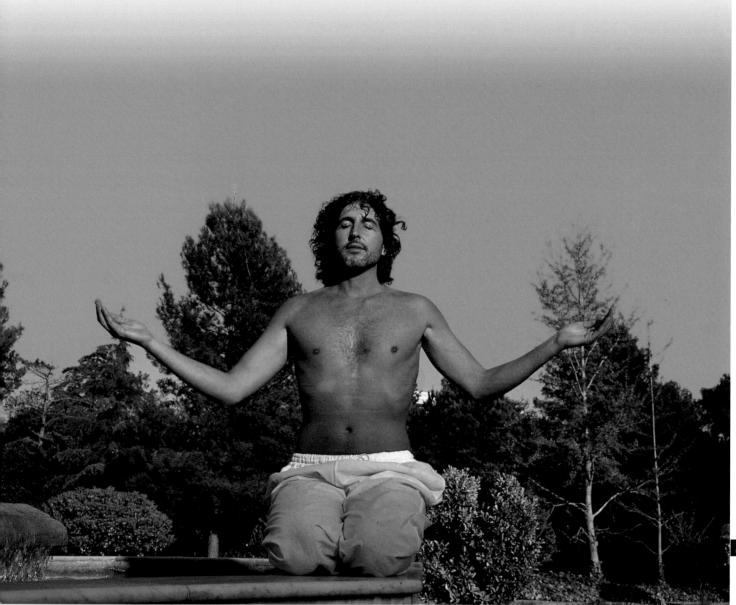

Pranayama is the key that allows you to unlock the chakras, activate them, and fill them with luminosity and power.

THE ART OF CONSCIOUS BREATHING

Respiration is our principle nourishment: although we can go thirty to forty days without eating, we can only hold our breath a few minutes.

The first thing we do after birth is breath, and throughout our life it becomes a vital subject, because our energy level depends on it. If we eat well in addition to breathing correctly, we will be in a state of perfect health.

But Tantra goes a little further, to transformation through energy.

Respiration is not connected to the past or the future, only the present. By breathing we can capture the eternal now.

Respiration is the thread that unifies the body, mind, and spirit.

An important fact (unknown in the Western world) about respiration is that it is not connected to the past or the future; respiration is always the present moment, and if you know that breathing and the mind are connected, you will focus both on the present and the now will be eternity.

By breathing you can capture the eternal instant! And the mind that is centered on the present is free of memories of the past and the worries of the future.

Because of this, Zen, Tantra, and Buddhism insist on the present and on breathing.

AWAKENING THE KUNDALINI

Adopt a comfortable meditation position (lotus, half lotus, or diamond) and breathe through the closed glottis, practicing breathing in three phases, which will produce a light snoring. You will note the current of air penetrate the trachea as a flow of prana; the flow of energy goes toward the heart and continues its path descending to the sexual center. Hold the breath and forcefully close the two sphincters, both external and internal. This is called the "root key" or mulabandha. You will feel that the tension has prolonged into the genital area, which stimulates the genital glands. Contract and relax the genital area and the sphincters, alternating various times, to activate the sexual center and to train the muscles of the genital region and intestines. The

Whoever masters the technique to awaken the kundalini, also awakens their inner master, with the possibility of conquering premature ageing and illnesses.

masculine member becomes erect, increases in size, and becomes excited because of the increased blood flow. The woman develops the ability to control vaginal muscles, increasing friction and excitation during contact with the member.

Thanks to the "root key," the apana is activated as opposing energy to the

THE THREE LOCKS

1. **Muladhara Bandha**
   Contraction of the anal sphincter.
2. **Uddinyana Bandha**
   Elevation of the abdomen.
3. **Jalandhara Bandha**
   Closing the throat. Lowering the chin to the chest.

THE FIVE FUNCTIONS OF PRANA

Respiration mobilizes the life force, prana. Through retention of breath, we master prana, and with exhalation, we apply its curative properties. The prana corresponds with the kundalini, which governs bodily, mental, and spiritual processes in dreams as well as during wakefulness.
In the organism it manifests:

▼ *As prana:*
Through inhalation, in the thorax region.

▼ *As apana:*
Through exhalation, in the lower abdomen, intestines, anus, and genital regions, where it controls the development of ovum and sperm cells, as well as orgasms and uterine contractions during birth.

▼ *As samana:*
In the stomach and the upper part of the abdomen, where it nourishes the furnaces of digestion and converts food to energy. It stimulates the harmonious function of the organs, the nervous system, and heart beat.

▼ *As udana:*
In the throat, controlling the process of swallowing and the mechanisms of speaking and singing, through the vocal chords.

▼ *Como vyana:*
Runs through the entire organism and orchestrates all the active forces, or vayu, via the circulatory system, maintaining erect posture of the body and also controlling decomposition after death.

prana. In this moment, lower the chin to the chest in jalandhara bandha and notice the flow of prana, manifested as a pressure that descends from the throat to the heart and then to the genital region. This exercise will lighten the cardiac work and there will be a slight lowering of blood pressure and heart rate. Here the pressure of the chin on the chest stimulates an acupuncture point that strengthens cardiac muscle. The clash of two opposing forces, apana and prana, produces a type of whirlwind of energy that intensely affects the genital region. Containing respiration now, lay your hands on your knees and tilt the chest lightly forward and pull in the navel as if you wanted to bring it back to the spine. This exercises is called "stomach key" or uddiyana bandha.

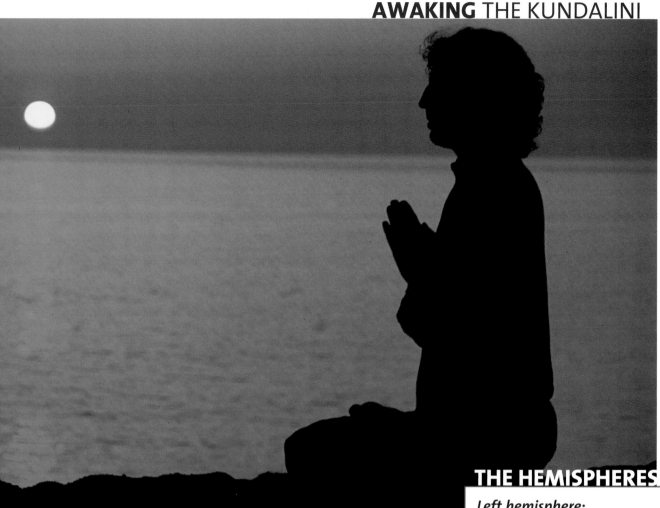

THE HEMISPHERES

Left hemisphere:
– Is critical
– Ruled by reason
– Is logical
– Is conscious
– Is local
– Controls words and intellect
– Has short term memory
– Sees only the tree and not the forest
– Calculates

Right hemisphere:
– The artist
– Ruled by intuition
– Is emotional
– Is subconscious
– Is holistic
– Controls symbols and images
– Has long term memory
– Sees the forest, and what is behind all actions
– Imagines, desires, and intuits
– Has fantasies
– Is wise

Lower the chin once more to the chest in jalandhara bandha and contract the sphincters. This combination is called the "great key" or maha bandha. Now you will feel an electric vibration like a hot ray of light running up along the central channel of the spine and ending in the third eye. All of the chakras activate through the tremendous passage of energy that charges all the cells. Repeat this exercise seven times. The second chakra corresponds with a center of the body called kanda, which is the point where all the subtle energetic channels of the astral body come together. The kanda is located level with coccyx and about five centimeters above the anus. From this center, the 72,000 subtle channels, the nadis, radiate out to the chakras and distribute energy through the whole physical and subtle bodies. The spiral force, kundalini, which unleashes the sensation of pleasure in the genital region, rests between the kanda and the root chakra. The mysterious force of kundalini awakens through this pressure directed toward the sexual center and kanda, which channels it and sends it toward the brain. Whoever masters this technique awakens their inner master and can conquer premature ageing and illnesses.

It is important to begin this exercise with the help of a yoga master.

PRANAYAMAS

1. NADI SODHANA
Polarized respiration of the Sun and the Moon

Inhale through the left nostril, plugging the right, and then exhale through the right, plugging the left, stop, repeat in the opposite direction. Inhale through the right, plugging the left, and then plug to the right and exhale through the left.
This is a complete cycle.

Benefits:
- Purifies the nadis
- Cleans and unplugs the nostrils
- Balances and stimulates the hemispheres of the brain
- Maintains health
- Prevents colds and improves digestion
- Activates sexual energy and helps control ejaculation
- Stimulates intellectual activities

Duration:
Ten minutes every morning and at sundown.

2. KAPALABHATI
"kapala"= "craneum"
"Bhati" = "to shine," "to clean"
Inhalation (puraka) for twice the time of the exhalation (rechaka) energetic and rapid.

Benefits:
- Cleans and purifies the lungs
- Charge the solar plexus with prana
- Stimulates the circulation and the throat
- Oncreases body temperature
- Saturates blood with oxygen
- Activates the chakras
- Strengthens abdominal muscles
- Benefits digestion
- Condition nervous system

- The inhalation lowers the volume of the brain and exhalation increases it
- Massages, pumps, and cleans the brain
- Revitalizes brain cells, activates pineal and pituitary glands
- Erases fatigue and toxins
- Eliminates lactic acid
- Combats asthma
- Refreshes the eyes
- Activates Ajna and Sahasrara chakras
- Prepares the mind for meditation
- Acts on the kundalini
- Incorporates more oxygen and eliminates carbon dioxide

The variation is called "bastrika" or "the bellows" and consists of inhaling and exhaling in the same beat and tempo. Here the most important part of breathing comes into play: retention or kumbhaka. By retaining the lungs full, we can have prana inside our bodies more time and close the bandhas.

Duration:
Start with two sets of 40 breaths (inhaling and exhaling counts as one), work up to three sets of 120 through practice. Between sets breathe completely and hold for five to ten seconds.

3. COMPLETE RESPIRATION
Covers the lower, middle, and upper parts. Works on the physical, emotional, and mental plane. Inhale, hold, and exhale for twice the time as inhalation. You can breathe counting mentally to seven to inhale, and twelve or fourteen to exhale.

Benefits:
- Activates circulation
- Benefits the heart (those with cardiac problems should not hold their breath)

- Activates and regenerates endocrine glands
- Develops will power
- Calms the mind
- By increasing prana it also increases intellectual and sexual energy
- Access the power of accumulated prana (psychic cures, transmission of energy, telepathy, premonitions, clairvoyance, los siddhis)
- Unites prana and apana
- Increases the electricity of the body in the energetic column and the chakras

Duration:
From five to twenty minutes

4. ABDOMINAL BREATHING
Inflate and deflate the abdomen like a child. Abdominal breathing is the first thing we do upon being born.

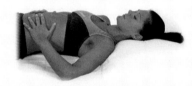

5. CIRCULAR BREATHING
Circular breathing or the tantric circle is a breath-meditation that dissolves the limits of the body and awakens energetic sensitivity. It is a breath that connects the inhalation and exhalation in the mouth, without space between them, performed in the same period of time. You can do it alone or with a partner, which awakens the bond between you two.

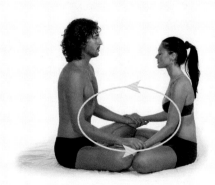

Benefits:
- Awakens the sensation of physical and spiritual unity
- Activates energy in the meridians
- Broadens the borders of the mind
- Prepares you to enter a deep meditation
- Provides peace and silence
- Leads to orgasm without penetration

Duration:
Twenty to forty minutes

6. CLEANSING BREATHING

With this practice, you clean stale energy out of your body and recharge with new prana, very useful if you've been with people with negative energy, or for living in a polluted environment (inevitable these days whether because of household appliances, smog, or automobile fumes).
Inhale through the nose and exhale through the mouth. The best posture is either shavasana or sidhasana.

Benefits:
- Cleanses the meridians
- Cleans and unblocks the solar plexus where heavy energies stagnate
- Charge the chakras with prana

Duration:
Ten to twenty minutes

7. RECHARGING RESPIRATION

Standing, legs squared with shoulders, breathe quickly and energetically, like a bellow in the nose, letting your body move from head to shoulders, arms, and hands, shaking as if you were covered in flour and wanted to get it off. Do this dynamically while breathing at the same quick rate. After five to ten minutes, stop and do seven complete breaths, visualizing your

whole body surrounded by light. You will obtain a very high level of energy for the rest of the day.

Benefits:
- Fills the nervous system with vital energy
- Activates the chakras and kundalini powerfully
- Cleans the nostrils
- Irrigates the brain with blood and prana
- Benefits memory
- Allows the physical body to maintain health and vitality without tiring

Duration:
Three to five minutes every day for the first week. Work up to ten minutes. There is no need to go any longer.

8. RESPIRATION FOR THE CHAKRAS

This is an important exercise to activate and cleanse the chakras. Inhale through the nose and exhale through the mouth, visualizing each chakra in its circular form and color. Do seven slow, deep breaths for each chakra. Continue in order, visualizing the colors red, orange, yellow, green, blue, white, and violet. Bring energy from the sexual pole to the brahamaranda, the site of the divine in the top of the head.

Benefits:
- Activates all the chakras, purifies and cleanses them, and elevates the kundalini

Duration:
Twenty to forty-five minutes. You can do three cycles, arriving at the seventh and starting over.

9. SURYA BREATHING
Solar respiration
Plugging the left nostril, inhale

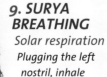

Observations:
Pranayama should be done at dawn or dusk, on an empty stomach. It's preferable to shower before to eliminate impurities, and to have an environment of concentration and comfort. Use a meditation posture with legs crossed or folded, but the most important is to keep the spine erect but not rigid. You can do it seated in a chair with the feet flat on the floor.

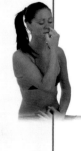

and exhale only through the right nostril, which is usually most active on Mondays, Tuesdays, and Saturdays, and during the dark half of the lunar cycle, waning and new.

Benefits:
- Activates the left hemisphere of the brain
- Warms the physical body

Duration:
Seven cycles.

10. CHANDRA BREATHING
Lunar respiration
Plugging the right nostril, inhale and exhale only through the left nostril. Normally respiration through the left nostril is strongest on Wednesdays, Thursdays, Fridays and Sundays, and when the Moon is bright.

Benefits:
- Activates the right hemisphere of the brain
- Refreshes the body and is good in the summer
- Affects the sympathetic nervous system and bodily functions
- Activates the influx of Shakti, the feminine principle

Duration:
Seven cycles.

71

DAILY PLAN

In the morning

1. Polarized breathing, 7 cycles
2. Recharging respiration, 10 minutes
3. Complete respiration, 7 cycles
4. Mahabhandas, 7 breaths with the "three locks"
5. Abdominal breathing, 3 minutes

Total time:
From 25 to 30 minutes

In the evening

1. Cleansing breathing, 10 minutes
2. Respiration for the chakras, 7 breaths for each
3. Circular breathing, alone or with partner, 15 minutes
4. Abdominal breathing, 10 minutes

Total time:
Approximately 45 minutes

You can vary the exercises depending on the phase of the moon. It is very positive to accumulate energy while the Moon is not visible to later (during waxing and full phases) practice maithuna and the visualization of a project intensely, or to reach a deeper state of consciousness. DON'T OVER DO IT with pranayamas, since they are very strong; it's best to start little by little, feeling the reactions you experience in your body and psyche. Remember that in nature nothing flowers in a day. Remember, too, that all energy is neutral: fire can warm you and illuminate the winter, but in excess, burn the forest. Water can slake your thirst or drown you. In the same way, pranayamas are useful in the right measure depending on how much you fill yourself with vitality. It's important to have a use for the energy planned, like something creative. If you follow the steps indicated, you will awaken your own inner master, but until then remain loyal to the instructions. Only people with arterial hypertension, ocular problems, or recent heart surgery patients should skip the pranaymas kapalabhati (recharging and for the chakras): for everyone else, they are fine.

MOON SALUTATION: *CHANDRA NAMASKA*

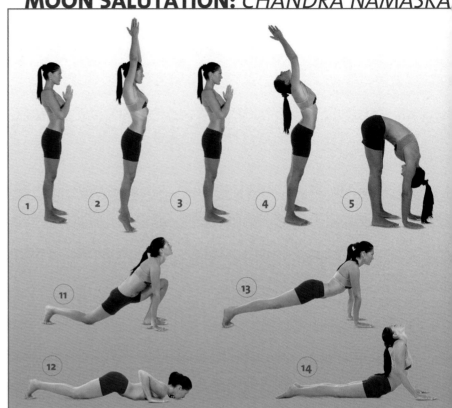

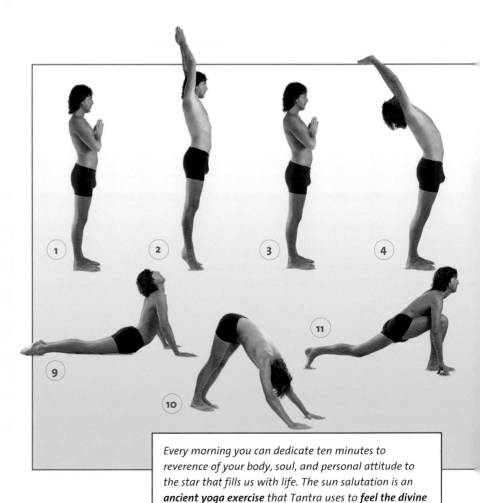

Every morning you can dedicate ten minutes to reverence of your body, soul, and personal attitude to the star that fills us with life. The sun salutation is an **ancient yoga exercise** that Tantra uses to **feel the divine presence** and to start the day with a flexible and vital body, as well as a good spiritual predisposition.

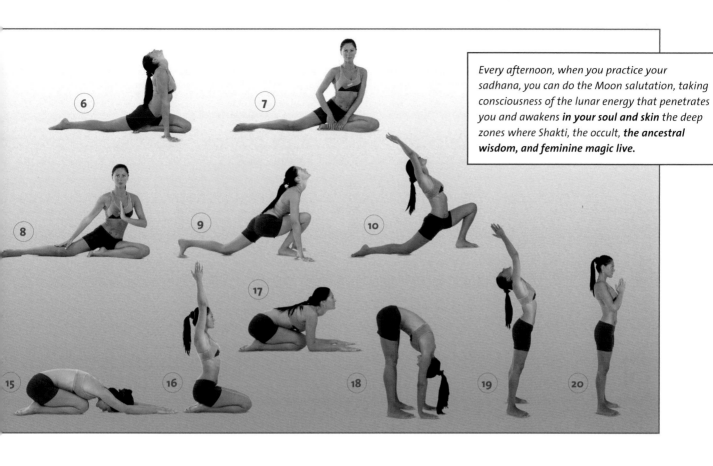

*Every afternoon, when you practice your sadhana, you can do the Moon salutation, taking consciousness of the lunar energy that penetrates you and awakens **in your soul and skin** the deep zones where Shakti, the occult, **the ancestral wisdom, and feminine magic live.***

SUN SALUTATION: *SURYA NAMASKAR*

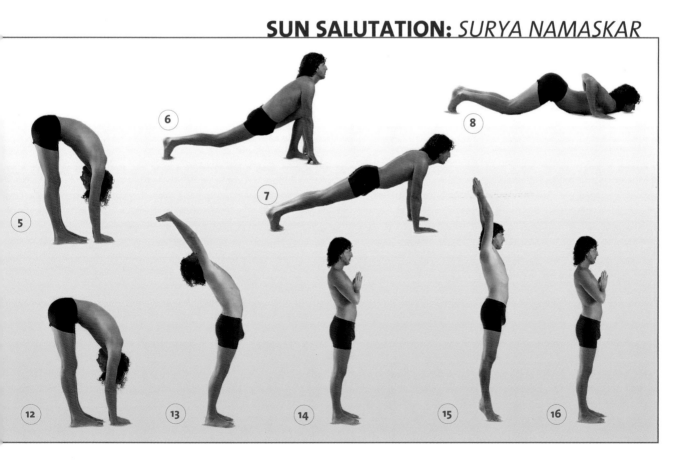

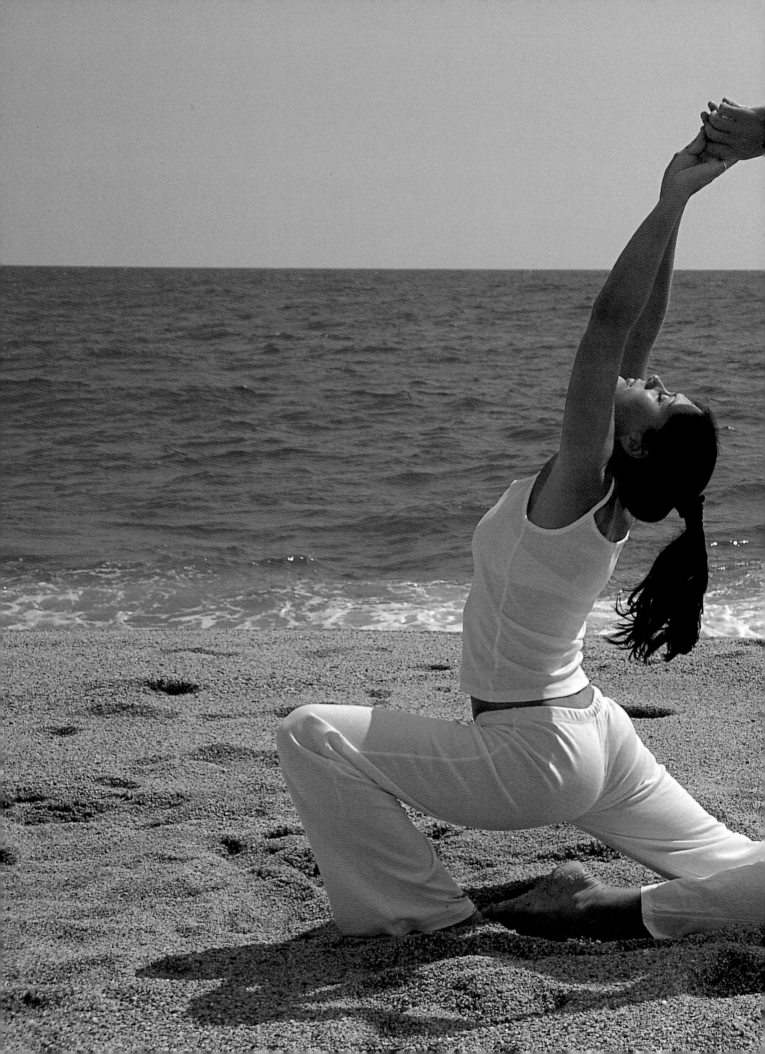

YOGA
IN PAIRS

*"He who knows the reality of his body
knows the reality of the universe."
Tantric principle*

HATHA YOGA:
Friend of Tantra

Yoga poses, or "asanas," have very precise effects on the body, mind, and emotions. Hatha Yoga, with its variety of techniques, allows you to achieve harmony and reach enlightenment.

Hatha Yoga is probably the method of Yoga most well known in the Western world. It is composed of an array of psychophysical and spiritual techniques to achieve harmony and Samadhi.

It consists of asanas, or poses of the body, that benefit energetic circulation in the meridians, stimulate the chakras, and release tension and stiffness from the musculature thanks to a high degree of flexibility. These poses are accompanied by a particular respiratory cadence and a mental state of silence.

The body is heard, valued, and prepared as if it were a dance hall ready for a party. As a temple, it is treated with love and care, so the postures (many referring to postures of animals) are practiced for their positive effects.

"Hatha Yoga" means "Yoga of the Sun and the Moon" (principles divided in the prefix "ha" and "tha") and its goal is the unity of polarities and the preparation of the body to receive the invited consciousness.

The asanas are determined bodily designs that tend to have precise effects on the body and its functions, character, energies, mind, and emotional system.

By mastering the body you achieve mastery over the mind. Each asana, or Yoga pose, requires the strict observation of a technique and some indispensible requirements, such as consistency, comfort, and stillness.

Yoga is the most ancient science of the human body in the world, so throughout history thousands of yogis have personally tested the benefits of each asana. Almost all of them are within reach of any person; you only need discipline without competition or being too fixated on a goal. There's no need to touch your forehead to your knee on the first try but stay conscious of caring for your body.

Although there are thousands of Yoga poses, there are only eighty-four traditional ones, and about twenty basic ones. These have been given

ASANAS: SOME ADVICE

Yoga poses require you to observe certain guidelines so that the changes—physical, mental, and energetic—happen correctly:

1. Breathe consciously and deliberately; mostly through the nose.

2. Maintain the posture at least 30 seconds and as much as 5 mintues.

3. Don't demand too much, on the physical plane or mental.

4. Enjoy the stretch without wanting to compete or "reach" a certain point.

5. Keep movements slow and gentle.

6. Don't practice asanas after eating; wait at least an hour.

7. Maintain consistency: take it as a sacred ritual.

8. Always keep your tongue on the roof of your mouth.

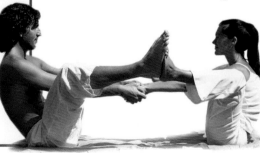

76

names of animals, plants, wise men, heroes, wizards, and divinities, or according to the characteristics of the particular asana.

POSES AND COUNTERPOSES

The spine is the axis of flexibility in the asanas. Therefore, in poses with posterior flexion remember that every time the spine goes backward we must compensate the movement with two poses with forward flexion. The vertebrae can acquire tremendous flexibility and elasticity with practice and you will enjoy seeing the results you get.

Asanas in partners allow you to do the pose and counterpose at the same time, since each partner does one and

Many tantric couples that regularly practice asanas awaken extrasensory abilities.

then the other. And since there are many postures, you can do two at once this way.

EXCHANGE OF ENERGY

By working in pairs, the chakras unite between two bodies, increasing tremendously the exchange of vitality and synchronization. Many tantric

couples that regularly practice asanas can awaken the siddhis or extrasensory abilities such as telepathy (knowing what the other is going to say and saying it at the same time), perception, intuition, and clairvoyance, which are symptoms of the opening of the higher chakras. The bioenergetic currents released by asanas in partners are a physical, amorous, and communicatory fuel for lovers.

NINETEEN BASIC POSES FOR COUPLES

1. The salutation

Seated face-to-face, with legs crossed in simple pose (sukhasana), half lotus (ardha siddhasana) or lotus (siddhasana), bring your hands to your chest signifying salutation and devotion to your partner with pranava mudra, the hand gesture. Look each other in the eyes, then close them and say "Namaste," which means "my soul greets your soul, since we are one."

In every tantric ritual or before each exercise or mediation, you will do this salutation (namaskar) which prepares your interior to take the act as sacred. It is Shakti greeting Shiva and the masculine greeting the feminine. Many couples have communication problems because they have lost or forgotten respect for the divinity they both possess.

Benefits:
Frees the mind from daily routine and trivial things. Connects the sadhakas with the divine vibration. Awakens the sacred consciousness and gives respect, profundity, and devotion to practice.

Duration:
One minute

Concentration:
In the center of the chest, anahata, chakra, the divine essence

Chakra stimulated:
Anahatta

2. The boat

Seated face-to-face approximately a yard apart, bend your legs and touch the soles of your feet together. Holding hands to maintain balance, lift your legs little by little until they are stretched fully. If you start to giggle, don't hold it back; but regain concentration quickly to feel the body.

Benefits:
Deeply stretches the legs, eliminating tiredness. Develops a better sense of balance. Remember that all asanas that offer physical balance also bring greater emotional and mental balance.

Duration:
Thirty seconds to a minute, undo and repeat three more times.

Concentration:
In the Third Eye, the base of the sacrum, and the abdomen

Chakra stimulated:
Ajna

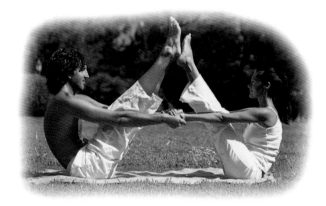

3. The half moon

Each partner bends their left leg forward and stretches the right leg out behind (later they switch). Stretch arms above the head and find your partner's hands. In this pose, the chest expands and the spine stretches back significantly, allowing the emotional chakras to open. It is a pose that gives great elasticity to the vertebrae and the act of finding each other up high gives both partners the sensation of elevation.

Benefits:
Opens the chest, the zone of sublime emotions. Stretches the abdomen. Stretches the spine and both legs.

Duration:
Fifteen to forty seconds. Repeat twice with each leg.

Concentration:
Spin, arms, and the support of the front foot

Chakra stimulated:
Anahatta and vishudda

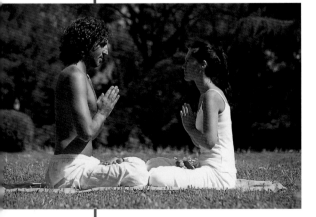

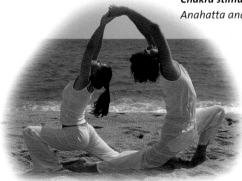

4. The swing

Standing back-to-back, link arms at the forearms. One remains immobile while the other leans forward and lowers their head to their knees. The other is lifted until their feet are off the ground. This asana produces a beneficial stability for both and is convenient when you are both of similar complexion. If the body weight remains well distributed, it is not difficult for the person on the bottom but helps them gain flexibility in the legs and back.

Benefits:
Stretches legs and spine considerably, as well as the meridians where prana flows through the body. Irrigates the brain with blood. Massages the stomach. Opens breathing for the person on top. Awakens the sensation of trust and confidence.

Duration:
One minute

Concentration:
In the legs and back for the person on the bottom; in the navel, center of chest, throat, and brow (yin line) of the person on top.

Chakra stimulated:
Manipura, anahatta, vishudda, and ajna

5. Lotus twist

Seated face-to-face with legs crossed and back straight, one person turns to one side and the other the opposite way. In this position, hold each other's forearms.

Benefits:
Allows for the rejuvenation of vertebrae. Massages the organs and intestines.

Duration:
Hold for 20 to 30 seconds, then change to the other side. Repeat three times.

Concentration:
In the thirty-three vertebrae of the spine, which is the tree of wisdom.

Chakra stimulated:
Although it's mainly an asana with physical effects, it also works on the manipura.

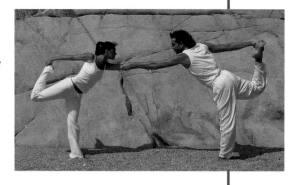

6. The dancer

Stand on one foot, take the other foot in one hand, and find your partner's outstretched arm with your free hand. It is a pose for balance that improves the circulation of prana between you. Look at a fixed point on the ground to keep you from falling, although if you do fall remember that "a fall is an invitation to get up and grow."

Benefits:
Generates balance in all aspects: physical, energetic, mental, and emotional.

Duration:
At least 1 minute

Concentration:
In the Third Eye

Chakra stimulated:
Ajna

79

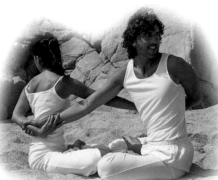

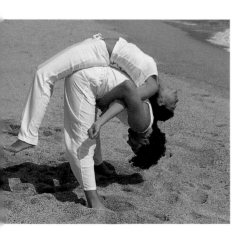

▼ Don't get down if your body is too stiff; practice is the only way to achieve flexibility.

▼ If you can't do an asana, go on to the next, but keep practicing until you can do it.

▼ Don't change the order of the asanas, it is designed to compensate the spine. Respect your body.

▼ Don't compare yourself to the models in the photos; if you practice you will get the same results. Give yourself permission to develop will and consistency. Just as reading bodybuilding magazines won't develop your muscles, observing the exercise without completing them doesn't help your body. Remember that the youth of the body is measured by the flexibility of the spine, not years.

▼ The duration of each asana is a suggestion, you can go longer if you feel comfortable.

*NOTE: People with hypertension, recent heart patients, and those with brain or gland problems should omit all inversion asanas.

NINETEEN BASIC POSES FOR COUPLES

7. The pyramid

Stand back-to-back with legs stretched as indicated in the photograph. Grab each other's forearms and lean forward without bending your knees. Exhale when you lower your torso and if have knee pain, bend them a little.

Benefits:
Stretches the legs. Massages the organs in the abdomen. Fully stretches the vertebrae, rejuvenating them. Recycles vital energy, allowing an increase in prana. Relaxes the neck and trapezeous muscles. Increases body heat. Stimulates kidneys and suprarenal glands.

Duration:
One to three minutes

Concentration:
In the first chakra, in the legs, and back

Chakra stimulated:
Muladhara, swadisthana, and manipura

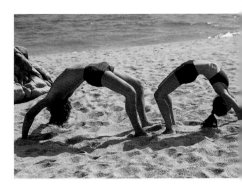

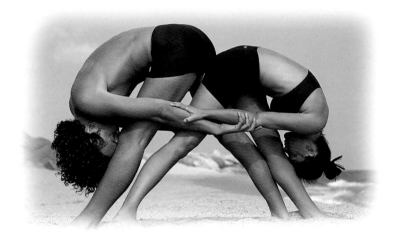

8. The clothespin

Sit facing each other with legs outstretched. Grab each other by the arms and lower your head to your knees, trying not to bend them.

Benefits:
Stretches legs and back. Massages organs in the abdomen. Irrigates the brain with blood, benefits the pineal and pituitary glands.

Duration:
Thirty seconds for each leg

Concentration:
In the base, using legs, arms, and spine to maintain balance

Chakra stimulated:
Ajna

9. The wheel

This asana requires practice and it's very helpful to have a partner to help you. You can do it separately. First, establish a proper base, with feet shoulder width apart. Inhale deeply and, stretching your arms over your head, bring your torso back until your hands reach the ground. Little by little, using the strength of your arms and legs, raise your torso until you form a semicircle. Your head should stay relaxed.

Benefits:
Stimulates all the endocrine glands and organs: gonads, suprarenal, kidneys, spleen, thyroid, parathyroid, pineal, and pituitary. Activates their complete function, which stimulates the psyche. Rejuvenates the vertebrae. Increases lung capacity. Strengthens arms and legs.

Duration:
Fifteen seconds to one minute

Concentration:
In the legs and vertebrae

Chakra stimulated:
All seven

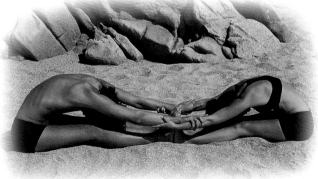

10. Fetal pose

Kneeling, with your forehead resting on the ground and arms stretched back, relax your spine, legs, and neck. Your partner gently climbs on top and you remain like twins. To think we spent nine months in this asana!

Benefits:
Completely relaxes the spine. Favors introspection. Increases spinal flexibility with the weight of another body.

Duration:
One to two minutes

Concentration:
In the whole spine

Chakra stimulated:
Muladhara, swadisthana, and manipura

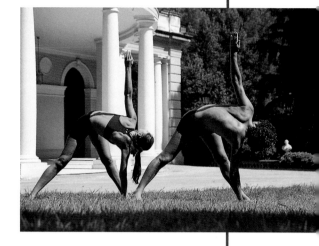

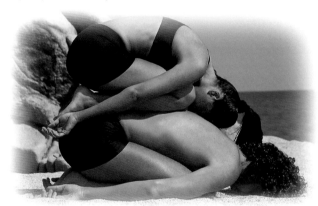

12. Parallel Triangle pose

Standing, separate your legs about a yard and lower your right arm to your left foot. Look at the opposite hand, which is stretched upward. Repeat with the other arm.

Benefits:
Stretches legs and vertebrae, rejuvenating them. Shrinks the waist and reduces excess weight in the belly area.

Duration:
Twenty seconds to a minute

Concentration:
In the legs and vertebrae

Chakra stimulated:
Manipura

11. The cobra

Lay face down and with hands on each side, lift your torso and lean your head back. The force should come from your arms, not your back.

Benefits:
Activates the kundalini. Deepens breathing. Stretches vertebrae and abdominal muscles. Strengthens arms.

Duration:
One to two minutes

Concentration:
In the first chakra and vertebrae

Chakra stimulated:
Muladhara and vishudda

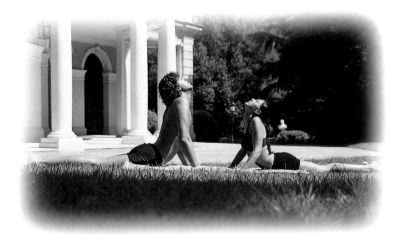

The Goraksashatakam says: "Everyone should turn to yoga, which is like the fruit of the Tree of Attained Desire. The yogi destroys sickness through poses; the karmas, through his control of breathing; and mental disturbances by retiring from the feelings of the external world. A yogi in the highest state of Samadhi is not affected by time or any other action."

NINETEEN BASIC POSES FOR COUPLES

13. The clothespin and the fish

One partner should sit with legs outstretched and hands on ankles, in the clothespin position. The other positions their back against their partner, forming a firm base with their legs. They then slide up until the napes of their necks are touching. Finally, they stretch their arms and hold the other's feet, in the pose of the fish.

Benefits:
In the clothespin: stretches legs, massages organs, completely stretches vertebrae, recycles vital energy allowing an elevation of prana, relaxes the neck and trapezeous muscles, increases body heat, stimulates kidneys and renal glands. In the fish: opens the chest and breathing, helps emotional openness, stretches the sacral area.

Duration:
One to three minutes

Concentration:
In the clothespin, in the first chakra, legs and vertebrae. In the fish, in the chest.

Chakra stimulated:
Muladhara, swadisthana, and manipura in the clothespin. Anahatta and vishudda in the fish.

14. The camel

With your genital areas touching, grab your own ankles to secure the base of this asana. The force should come from your arms and legs, never from the spine or sacrum.

Benefits:
Opens the solar plexus, heart, and throat chakras, as well as deepening lung capacity. Improves blood flow to the brain and relaxes the neck.

Duration:
Twenty seconds to one minute

15. The headstand and the tree

It's best to start practicing "the headstand" or shirsasana with the help of your partner. First make a triangle with hands interlaced, then rest the top of your head between them. Rest your head on the ground and lift first one leg, then the other. It's best if the other person is behind you, which also helps psychologically with the fear. If you situate the head properly, there's no risk to the cervical vertebrae, and once you get the hang of it, you'll never want to come down!

"The tree," or vakrasana, is a balance pose where you stand on one leg and rest the other against the thigh. At the same time, lift your arms above your head with palms together. Keep your eyes on a fixed point on the ground at a 45∞ angle.

Benefits:
Of "the headstand": Activates the endocrine glands, improves memory, improves blood flow to brain, transmutes sexual energy into ojas shakti, strengthens arms, generates control of the body and mind, recycles vial energy, improves immune defenses, eliminates tiredness, clears the mind, relaxes the heart beat, opens the breathing capacity, massages the organs and intestines, rejuvenates the body by receiving energy in the opposite direction—prana through the feet and apana through the head. Of "the tree": Strengthens physical, mental, and emotional balance, develops intuition and works the Third Eye, strengthens legs, deepens breathing, generates a pleasant feeling of stability, introspection, and mental balance.

Duration:
Fifteen seconds to five minutes

Concentration:
In "the headstand": the whole spine and the feet (since you have to keep them in line). In "the tree": the Third Eye.

Chakra stimulated:
All seven

Concentration:
In the lumbar area

Chakra stimulated:
Anahatta

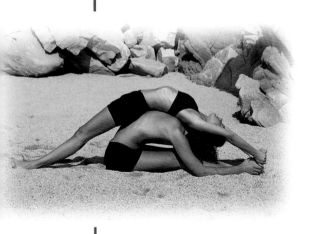

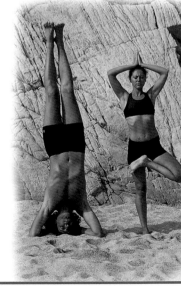

16. The candle

Laying face up, bring your knees to forehead while placing your hands firmly on your lumbar region. Lift your legs, together and outstretched, little by little. You can play a little with the leg position to avoid pressure on your neck; it's more important to be comfortable than how it looks.

Benefits:
The same as "the headstand," except this sends more blood to the throat, which benefits the thyroid and creative chakra.

Duration:
Thirty seconds to five minutes

Concentration:
In the lumbar region and legs

Chakra stimulated:
Mostly Vishudda, but also Ajna

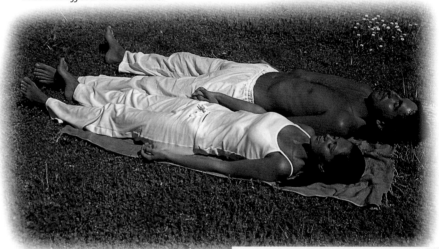

17. The candle with diamond

Variation of "the candle" or sarvangasana, with the soles of the feet touching. Rests the legs and improves knee flexibility. This asana has practically the same effects as the candle.

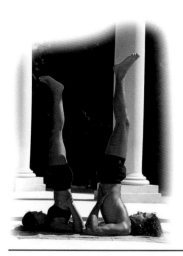

18. Child's pose

A restful pose. Stretch your hands over your head, relaxing the spine and neck. Favorable for introspection and the gate to relaxation and meditation.

Benefits:
Helps you to take consciousness of the state of your body and mind.

Duration:
Undetermined

Chakra stimulated:
Calms the affect of previous work

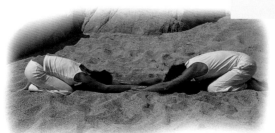

19. Corpse pose, or Yoga nidra

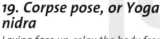

Laying face up, relax the body from head to feet, seeking to sink into the feeling of total lightness. You will be more energy and less material. Many practitioners experience an out-of-body experience, or "astral journey," because the body experiences a strong receptiveness to new energy and this circulates through the chakras through consciousness. Don't be afraid and don't hang onto the physical body; let it happen, let it flow. When you reach this point, relax and enjoy. The mind will be silent and consciousness will expand without limit.

83

FINAL RELAXATION

After the sequence of asanas, lay in shavasana, breathe softly and abdominally, and relax one by one all the muscles of the body, from head to toes. After a few minutes, you will enter a profound state of relaxation, pleasure, and consciousness, perceiving your body as floating energy. Let your consciousness deepen in the silence and peace.

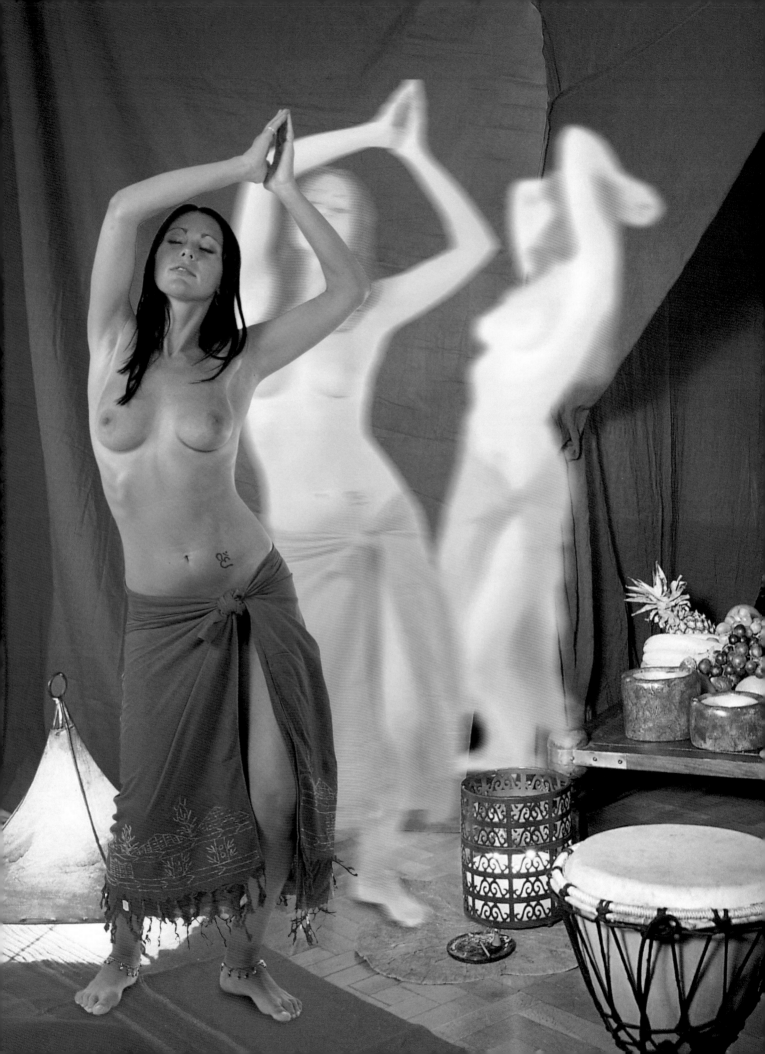

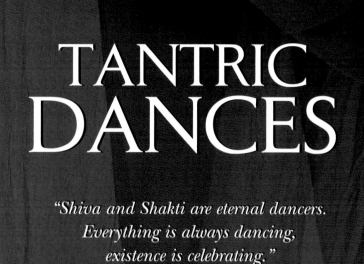

TANTRIC DANCES

*"Shiva and Shakti are eternal dancers.
Everything is always dancing,
existence is celebrating."*

THE DANCE
of the Universe

Daily tensions can cause huge energy blockages. With dance,
we not only can relax, but also connect with nature and transcend
consciousness on a deeper level.

Tantra seeks movement in everything: in the planets that dance around the sun; in the trees that dance in the wind; in the Earth, a circle of energy in motion; in the waves, hips of an ocean that dance endlessly . . . Even in human beings, that surround themselves with music and for whom dance is intimately related to celebration since the dawn of time.

In tantric sadhana, dancing is the first step to opening and awakening the vital energy of the body. Modern men and women accumulate stress and tension in different areas, causing huge energetic blockages.

Tantric dance isn't a popular dance, and it has nothing to do with the moves you see in the club. Tantric dance is a meditative practice to free the soul, increase vitality, connect to the consciousness in deep trance states, and to improve the body.

Dance was the first of the arts; a curative art that ancient shamans and masters, from Australia to Mexico, India to Africa, have used as a means of transcending ordinary consciousness to a deeper vibratory level. But dance also connects the dancer with the forces of nature: with the stones, the plants, the animal spirits, and the enlightened human soul. When a tantric dances, they become an antenna between the sky and the earth, an instrument to celebrate the presence of life in the cells, the blood, the brain, the muscles, and the chakras.

In ancient times, some tribes used ritual dances to cure illnesses, to ask for fertility or bountiful harvests, or to have a healthy birth.

In the last case, women danced, sang, and waited for the new being with total happiness, with the future other dancing with them until the

PRINCIPLES OF TANTRIC DANCE

Tantra uses dances as a way to reach catharsis, cleansing, and purification of emotions, energy that doesn't flow, and tense minds. Tantric dance is a bridge to dancing with life, where divisions disappear and you will feel complete unity. Flexibility is the first sign that Tantra is becoming part of you; not just in your physical body but in your character as well.

In tantric dance you leave behind control, shame, and repressions, which allows for liberation of new and higher emotions.

Dance is a means of connection between the individual heart and nature, the five elements. It's possible to feel the abundance of the earth through your feet, the fluidity and depth of the water, the enthusiasm and creativity of fire, the freedom of the air, and the silence and lightness of ether. By dancing we break internal barriers that have nothing to do with intellectual processes. You can transform depression into celebration, fear into enthusiasm, rigidity into flexibility. The body becomes energy, and we cease to feel like material. The individual name is almost forgotten because the universe and power of nature dance through the transpersonal human.

86

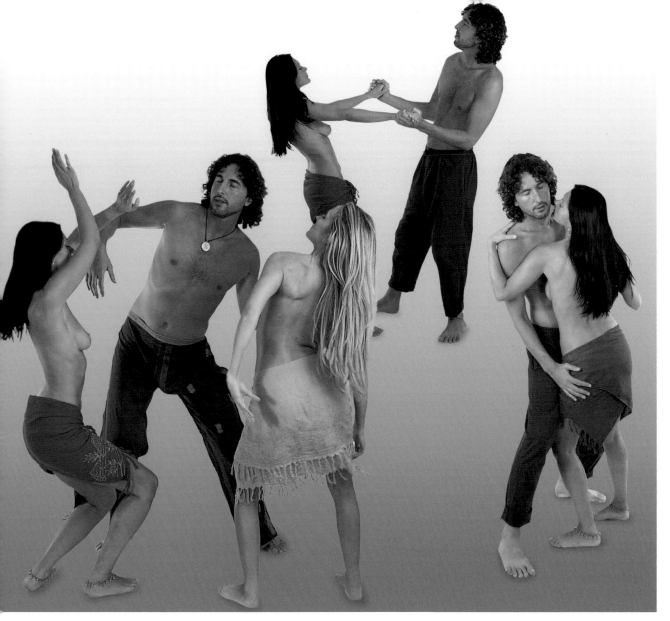

The dances that Tantra offers are more than just simple dances; they are authentic meditations in motion.

moment she gave birth. What a big difference to come into the world with your mother dancing than to do it in a hospital, where they cut the umbilical cord and you are blinded by bright lights.

INSTRUMENT OF CONSCIOUSNESS

In transformation, the consciousness expands and this leads to ecstasy.

Dance is the best form of dynamic meditation for modern men and women to unleash their inner god or goddess, as well as to openly experience their latent and creative potential.

> Dance opens the consciousness and awakens eroticism, which is the expression of the joy of living.

Almost all the dances of the ancient times come from ethnic or tribal rituals in honor of gods or natural forces; the majority were meant to obtain material goods, spiritual powers, and alterations of the ordinary consciousness. However, western religious traditions

(especially Christianity) have prohibited for centuries the rituals and dances that adored the feminine part of God. This has conditioned the body and soul, since it has kept people away from contact with the magic forces of nature.

Dance doesn't only open the consciousness, but also awakens the eroticism and sensuality of energy in the body, which is the expression of the joy of living.

The dances also allow the shedding of accumulated layers of repression, through catharsis and breathing.

MAGIC DRUMS

When a woman moves her hips in figure eights, her torso and neck undulates, her hair swings sensually, and her arms move (along with her body) to the rhythm of the drums or the magnetic sound of a flute, she is connected to her interior and bringing the best of herself to the surface.

The drums envelope the dancer, whether man or woman, in a strange connection to the rest of the universe. As the proverb says: "In her hips, the stars move."

Meditative dance involves the whole body. Blood, for example, pulses inside you to the beat of the drums; the fire element grows and spiritual impulse emerges. The drum and the didgeridoo are the most ancient ancestral instruments of humanity. They have a hypnotic power on the mind and thoughts, and they are a means to clearly perceive hidden aspects of nature.

TO BREATHE AND TO FEEL

In the Tantra seminars I teach, I put a special emphasis on the slogan "to breathe and to feel," since it is through breathing you renew energy and eliminate tension. Breathing, along with meditative consciousness and sensitivity, is a fundamental pillar so that the dances have maximum effect.

When you dance, you breath as a means of increasing spiritual combustion. Just as air stokes the fire, breathing consciously kindles the spirit.

If you don't allow the mind to interfere with thoughts or worries, breathing will keep you in the present moment, which is its great importance and link to the eternal.

1. DANCE OF THE TANTRIC PRINCIPLES

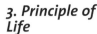

With a partner
Duration: *About 45 minutes (3 minutes to start)*
Objective: *To feel the principles of life in the human body*

1. Principle of Unity

Standing, hands clasped, face-to-face with eyes closed and breathing in the same rhythm, you will begin to fuse with the music and feel the original principle of cosmic unity.

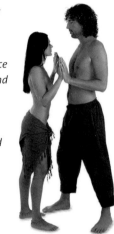

2. Principle of Contraction and Expansion

Still holding hands, begin moving back, exhaling through the mouth, then go forward again until your foreheads are touching, inhaling through the nose; a swaying motion that personifies on a small scale the movement of the universe.

3. Principle of Life

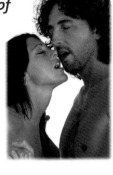

You will emphasis the principle of life with soft movements and by feeling your breath and the breath of your partner. Inhale through the nose and exhale audibly through the mouth with an "Ahhahhahhhahh."

4. Principle of Creation and Dance

The universe is the dance of Shiva with which the planets move around the Sun. Now dance with your partner back-to-back, still holding hands, to feel the fire from your sacrum upward, to the sound of a special music.

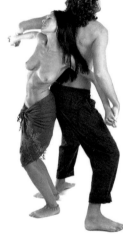

BENEFITS OF TANTRIC DANCE

▼ *Balances you emotionally*
▼ *Reinforces your confidence in yourself*
▼ *Softens facial and bodily expressions*
▼ *Releases deep tension*
▼ *Brings happiness and wellbeing to your daily life*
▼ *Elevates the kundalini*
▼ *Corrects poor posture, reducing back pain and tension in the shoulders*

▼ *Unblocks the genital area, improving sexual satisfaction*
▼ *Helps in birthing or menstruation*
▼ *Awakens spiritual power*
▼ *Increases creativity and enthusiasm*
▼ *Silences the mind quickly*
▼ *Deepens breathing*
▼ *Connects you with Creation*
▼ *Fine tunes intuition, freedom, and joy*
▼ *Strengthens the soul*

5. Principle of Pleasure

Give each other subtle caresses with your hands, breathing deeply and slowly at all times to circulate energy through the body. Touch each other freely with sandalwood, cinnamon, almond, or jasmine oils. The body will feel pleasure all over, feeling more like energy than material. In this principle, it's important to start eliminating areas with repressions and taboos, freeing the chakras.

6. Principle of Love

With gentle movements, bring your right hand to your partner's chest and your left hand to the center of their back, at the heart chakra. Breathe in the same rhythm and feel their heartbeat and the heat of their hand flooding your chest with love. The man will feel devotion for his Shakti, and the woman, for her Shiva.

7. Principle of Desire

The contact will increase in intensity, until your bodies are interlaced in an erotic and exciting dance. Your desire will grow, but always maintain the consciousness of an observer. Intense touches, hugs, and caresses on your body will make the desire, fire, and passion mix in complete freedom.

TANTRIC INSTRUCTIONS FOR DANCING

1. *Breathe consciously*
2. *Disconnect the mind*
3. *Free all the areas of the body, especially the pelvis, neck, and head*
4. *Put your whole being into the dance*
5. *Feel the kundalini and elevate it*
6. *Open yourself to experience the divine*
7. *Let the movement carry you to stillness, and the music take you to silence*

8. Principle of Giving and Receiving

Standing, hands clasped and eyes closed, give each other loving caresses and fine energy through your hands. Balance giving and receiving.

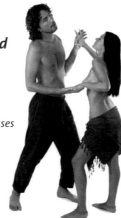

9. Principle of Peace

After building up desire, you will stop moving and enter progressively into a state of peace and calm. Just as before you were building the fire, now you will distribute it freely through your body, connected spiritually in peace and joy. At this point, everything is filled with a calm and subtle connection.

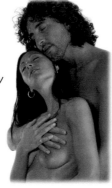

10. Principle of Birth

In this principle we change position: facing each other in child's pose, back-to-back (like the seed of a new man and woman), you will connect through the chakras and breathe softly into a deep state.

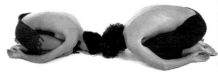

11. Principle of Silence and Nothingness

Lay on your side, the man to the right of the woman. Face-to-face, look each other in the eyes a few seconds; then, eyes closed, elevate yourself internally to silence and nothingness. You will feel ecstasy, communion, innocence, and connection, going from the exciting to the profound, from the body to the luminous soul, like a spiritual staircase that goes from the dense to the sublime accepting each plane with love and freedom.

*After doing all the dances, **relax for fifteen minutes in shavsana.***

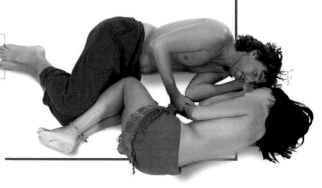

PRACTICES

2. DANCE OF ENERGY, SEATED

With a partner
Duration: *From 30 to 45 minutes*
Objective: *Connect the bioenergies between bodies*

Sit in meditation and keep your legs still. Grasp each other's hands and let your torsos move with the sound of the music. Breathe and feel the currents of energy passing from one to the other. The movement should be free.

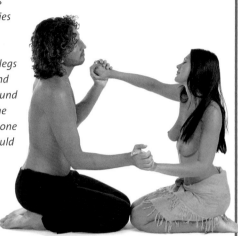

4. DANCE OF THE CH

Individual
Duration: *45 minutes*
Objective: *To cleanse and energize the chakras*

Connecting to a special music for each chakra, you will move the part of the body that corresponds to each while performing a cleansing breath. The sound, the movement, and the breathing will make the energy go step by step through the plexus and eliminate barriers and psychoemotional defenses. By mobilizing the body, you move emotions and psychological resistance.

3. DANCE OF THE FIVE ELEMENTS

Individual
Duration: *45 minutes*
Objective: *Connect with the earth, the water, the air, the fire, and the ether*

Just as they did in tribal rituals, strike the ground with your heels to activate the first chakra. This mobilizes the earth element, related with abundance and earthly power.
    The water element you will awaken with broad, undulating movements aimed at the second chakra. Later, with movements that open the

arms and the chest, the air element and fourth chakra will awaken. The passion, spirit, enthusiasm, and inner luminosity will be present in you through the sound of the drums, which activate the fire element in the third chakra. Finally, lay on the ground in complete silence, feeling the connection and deep relaxation. Work on each element for about seven minutes.

Earth: *Benefits the contact between the psyche and the material and*

economic aspect; the roots of the being.

Water: *Frees sensitivity and the delicate emotional states.*

Air: *Unleashes the sensation of freedom, openness, and immensity.*

Fire: *Increases spiritual power, strength, and will power.*

Ether: *Laying in silence.*

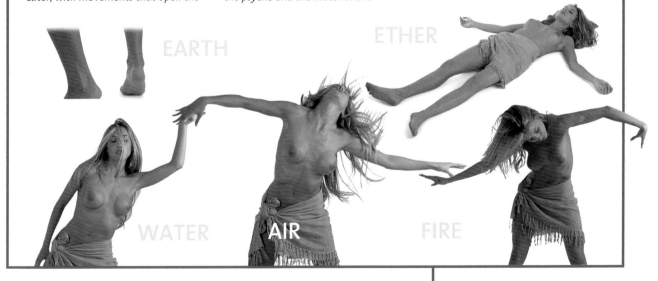

EARTH ETHER WATER AIR FIRE

Movements for the chakras:

First
Rotation of the pelvis forward and back in a figure eight. The heels connect to the ground.

Second
Erotic and sensual movements of the genital area, as if you were making love.

Third
Widening of the solar plexus, balance of the center of the body. Deepen the cleansing breaths.

Fourth
Movements that open the arms and chest, like an eagle in flight.

Fifth
Soft unblocking with slow, sensual rotation of the neck, trapezius, and head.

Sixth
Dance with all the parts of the body moving freely, focusing energy in the Third Eye.

Seventh
Let the gentle dance connect you to everything that flows. Without mind or time, the energy is what moves.

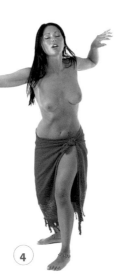

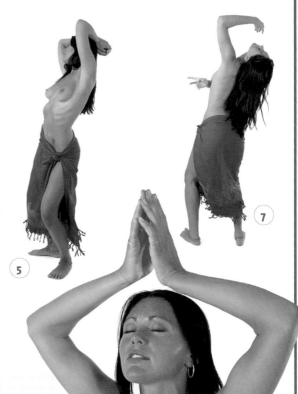

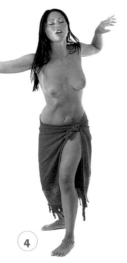

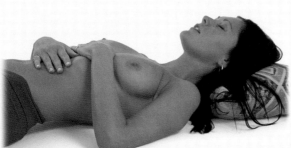

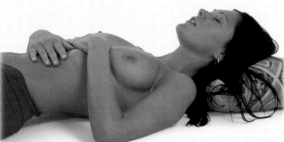

91

After periods of each chakra, lay face up for fifteen minutes and enjoy the feeling of peace and energetic envelopment.

6. **DANCE** OF THE BUDDHA

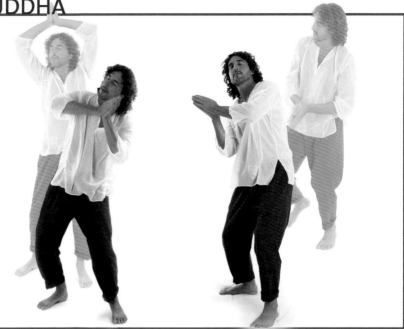

Individual
Duration: *15 to 20 minutes*
Objective: *Tune in to your inner Buddha*

Connect yourself with your center in solitude and silence. Meditate on something nice that has happened to you recently, or on the emptiness, the infinite, the universe, or the mystery of life. Once you have this mental image, dance gently, later increasing the rhythm as you feel the strength of Buddhist love inside you. Finish celebrating and enjoying your life.

5. **DANCE** OF SHIVA AND SHAKTI

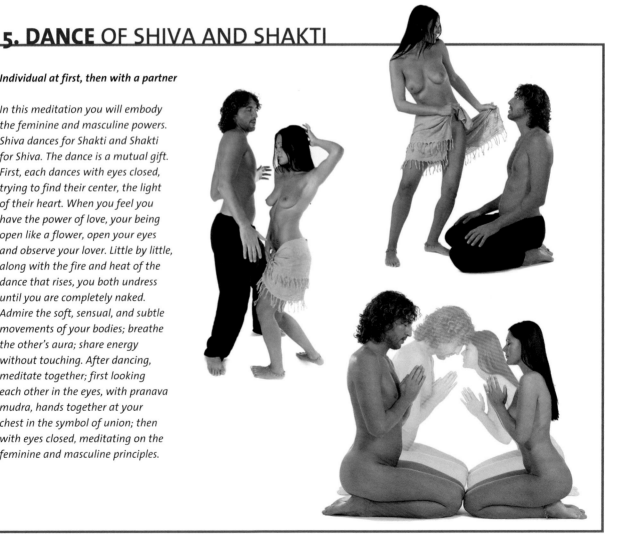

Individual at first, then with a partner

In this meditation you will embody the feminine and masculine powers. Shiva dances for Shakti and Shakti for Shiva. The dance is a mutual gift. First, each dances with eyes closed, trying to find their center, the light of their heart. When you feel you have the power of love, your being open like a flower, open your eyes and observe your lover. Little by little, along with the fire and heat of the dance that rises, you both undress until you are completely naked. Admire the soft, sensual, and subtle movements of your bodies; breathe the other's aura; share energy without touching. After dancing, meditate together; first looking each other in the eyes, with pranava mudra, hands together at your chest in the symbol of union; then with eyes closed, meditating on the feminine and masculine principles.

7 TO ELEVATE THE KUNDALINI

Individual
Duration: 20 minutes
Objective: Lift the sacred energy along the spine

This dance is done with the music of drums and the didgeridoo, and is especially powerful. The intruments make the vibration and movement awaken your life energy. At the beginning, you can strike your heels on the ground to stimulate the first chakra. Once you feel a tickle in the sacrum, imagine that the energy is orange and that it rises along the central channel (sushumna) up to the head and mixes with the energy of the universe. Visualize how this divine mixture of energy falls like rain over your body, entering your skin, cells, organs, and chakras. Breathe consciously at all times and release the tension from your body so that energy becomes liquid. Finally, finish laying in shavasana.

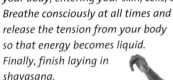

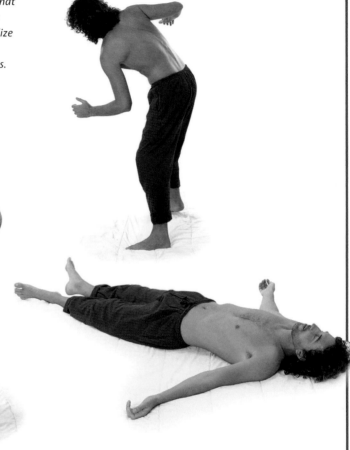

8. DANCE OF THE TIGER

Individual
Duration: 15 to 20 minutes
Objective: To awaken inner power

The tigress is the one that hunts her prey, so this is a feminine and powerful dance, for women as well as the feminine part of men. Imitating the stealthy, soft, and alert movements of the tiger, you will move your body and arms, dancing as if you were in a fertile valley. It is a very soft dance that imitates the movements and leaps of the cat: feel the mystery of animal instinct and its power. Moving the body, breathing, and visualizing the embodiment of the feline in your being, you will fill your heart with fire and light.

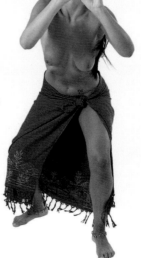

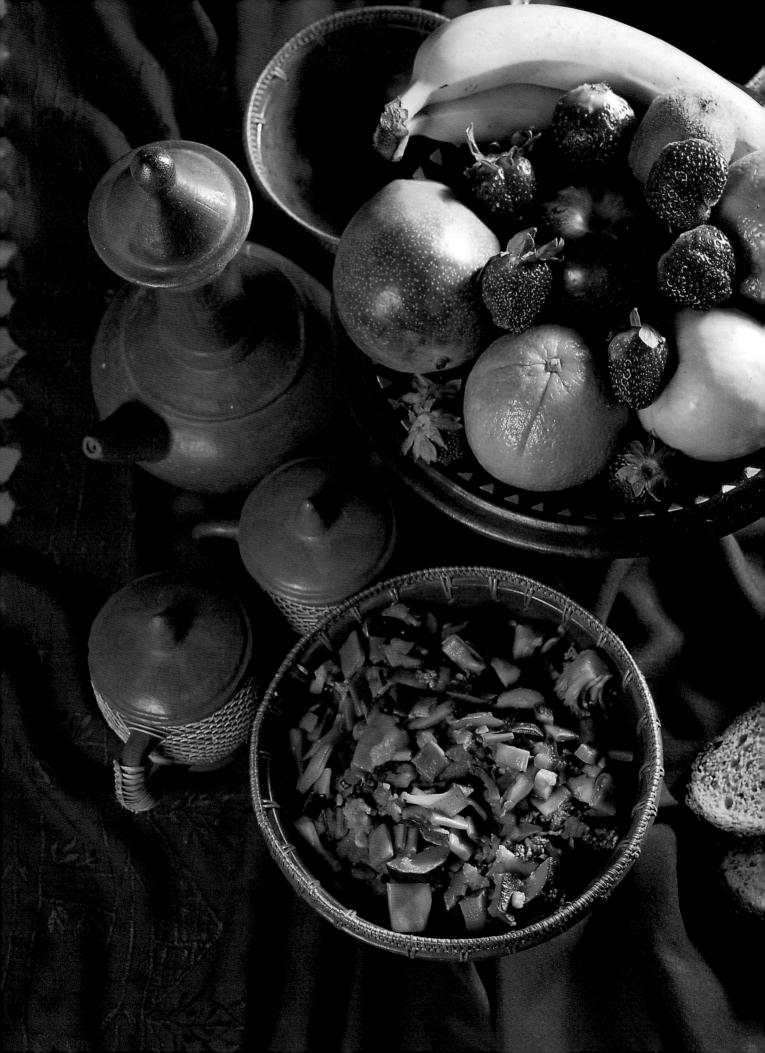

TANTRIC
FOOD

"Let food be thy medicine."
Hippocrates

INTELLIGENT
Eating

For Tantra, choosing the right foods is fundamental for good

health in body and spirit. In order to eat intelligently,

you must know the properties of

what you eat and when to eat them.

Nutrition isn't so much what we eat but what we digest. A healthy and balanced diet makes for healthy and generous individuals, while malnutrition or overeating produces negative people. Therefore, an intelligent diet is not only good for bodily health but also for that of the spirit, since both form an integrated and indivisible whole.

To achieve an intelligent and balanced diet, you must keep in mind the properties of what you eat—know which foods are yin and which are yang, and when to eat them. The yin and yang principles are two opposites that complement each other, with yin representing cold and negative, and yang, warm and positive. An energetic diet should have, in general, similar quantities of both elements.

But, depending on the season or your mood, you can eat more foods of one polarity.

In the cold months, it's recommended you eat more yang foods, since their warm qualities balance your diet, while in warmer months you should eat more yin foods, whose cold properties are ideal for summer. If you find yourself sad or depressed, yang foods are recommended, while yin foods are fine if you are in an optimistic and energetic state.

Tantric nutrition is not just limited to dividing foods in yin and yang, but also about modifying life style for a healthier diet.

FUNDAMENTAL RULES

1 Don't eat artificial foods that contain colorants or preservatives.

2 Avoid refined foods such as flour, rice, and white sugar; eat whole grains instead.

3 The ideal foods are those native to your area and that are in season. Your environment provides all the necessary elements for a good diet.

4 Food should be chewed thoroughly (at least forty times) to be easily digested.

5 It is important to eat only when you're hungry; if we continually fill ourselves with food, the body cannot assimilate and accumulates toxins.

6 You shouldn't eat before going to sleep.

7 The atmosphere where you eat is very important, and should be peaceful and pleasant.

THE DANGER OF DIETING

For Tantra, all repression is poisonous, and a forced diet makes you eat foods you don't want. Eat what you want if you feel that you need to; just remember that if you consume more calories than you spend, you will end up accumulating them in the form of fat. But if one day you eat too many calories, don't feel guilty; enjoy them knowing that later you'll do your sadhana and maintain your weight that way.

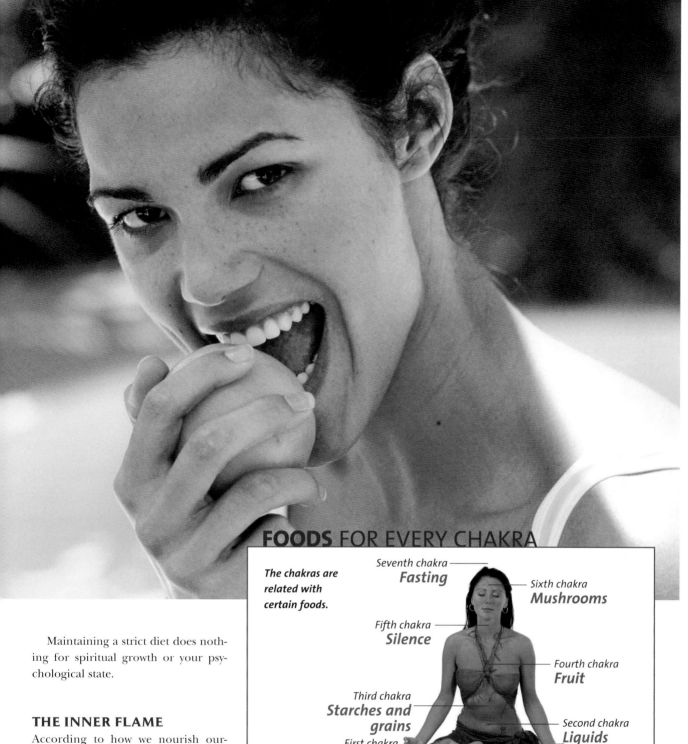

FOODS FOR EVERY CHAKRA

The chakras are related with certain foods.

Seventh chakra
Fasting

Sixth chakra
Mushrooms

Fifth chakra
Silence

Fourth chakra
Fruit

Third chakra
Starches and grains

Second chakra
Liquids

First chakra
Fish and proteins

Maintaining a strict diet does nothing for spiritual growth or your psychological state.

THE INNER FLAME

According to how we nourish ourselves, so will be the flame we generate in our interior.

We have to invest time in reflecting on how we feel ourselves, since from this we derive good blood quality, strengthened immune system, higher energy, lucid intellect, and an active will. It is necessary to choose biological, healthy, and natural foods; like fruit, dry as well as fresh, which we should eat at intervals throughout the day. Remember that the body already knows what foods it needs; for example, on cold days we tend to eat hot, high energy foods, while in summer we crave fruit and salads. If you feel you inner flame is low, active foods, breathing, and dances help lift your mood.

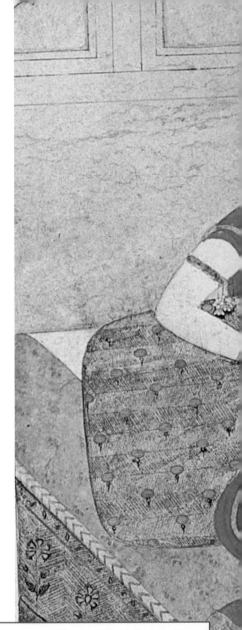

YANG FOODS

salt • crustaceans • miso
pescado blanco • huevos •
white fish · eggs •
lettuce · endive
radish • garlic • onion
parsley lentils • goat's milk
cherries • buckwheat
carrots
apples • chicory

YIN FOODS

lard
olives
oils • water
raw • sugar
vinegar •
vegetables alcoholic
beverages • fruit milk • cheese
seaweed • rye • beets • oysters •
clams • peanuts • corn
yogurt • octopus
thyme • mint · menta
almonds • hazelnuts
mushrooms

New dieticians agree with oriental traditions that grains are the most balanced foods.

YIN AND YANG FOODS

Each food corresponds with an energetic principle: yin is feminine, cold, receptive and light, while yang is masculine, hot, active, and energetic. It is important to know how to combine foods not only for a balanced diet but also for a good relationship, since the poles appear clearly in couples: if a woman vibrates in yin because she eats those foods, and her partner in yang, this generates mutual attraction. But if the woman convinces her husband to be vegetarian and stop eating yang foods, the attraction will probably diminish, and the same the other way around. What one eats is the energy that later manifests on the exterior.

It's important to eat some foods that your partner doesn't. For example, if the man eats fish (yang), the woman should eat vegetables (yin), and so on, combining yin and yang so that both feel energetically attracted. However, as Jesus said, "What's important is not what goes in the mouth, but what comes out." Tantra maintains that love is the most important food, and everything else only helps this fire grow.

GUIDE TO EATING WELL

1. Chew your food well:
It is the best way to save the digestive system unnecessary effort. Also, it helps achieve a feeling of fullness without eating too much.

2. Eat meditatively:
Dedicate all your attention to the pleasurable act of eating. The digestive system reacts to sates of stress, worry, or irritation, and doesn't function well.

3. Savor and enjoy:
Take note of what you are eating and fine tune your ability to differentiate flavors: what tastes good to you will surely sit well.

4. Eat fresh fruit between meals:
Fruit is very healthy, since it provides many vitamins with few calories, so it is ideal for a snack between meals.

5. Don't eat to fullness:
You need to leave the table with a light sensation of hunger. Eating moderately lengthens your life, and that of your intestines and stomach.

6. Eat a varied diet:
It is the best way to make sure you don't lack nutrients. Take advantage of the variety in the market, with preference to foods that are in season.

7. Drink if you are thirsty:
It isn't true that you can't drink during meals because it dilutes digestive juices. Although it's true that the more natural your diet, the less thirsty you'll be, you can drink a little wine with meals.

8. Make simple dishes:
It's not necessary to make meals with sauces or strong condiments.

9. Breakfast like a king, lunch like a prince, and dine like a pauper:
This is the perfect distribution of meals as far as quantity. In the morning we should charge ourselves with energy, and eat little at night to not overload the digestive system.

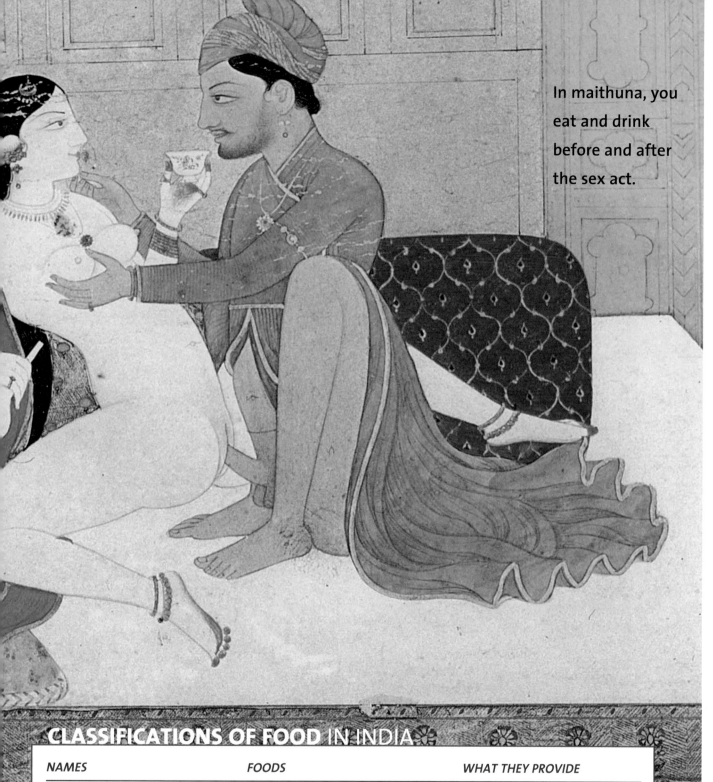

In maithuna, you eat and drink before and after the sex act.

CLASSIFICATIONS OF FOOD IN INDIA

NAMES	FOODS	WHAT THEY PROVIDE
SATTVA	Fruits (dried and fresh), vegetables, honey, and milk.	Provide clarity, lightness, and purity.
RAJAS	All meats, eggs, and onions.	Provide passion, activity, and coarseness
TAMAS	Preserves, artificial and industrially processed foods.	Related to darkness and laziness

TANTRIC RECIPES FOR MAITHUNA: THE FOODS OF THE GODS

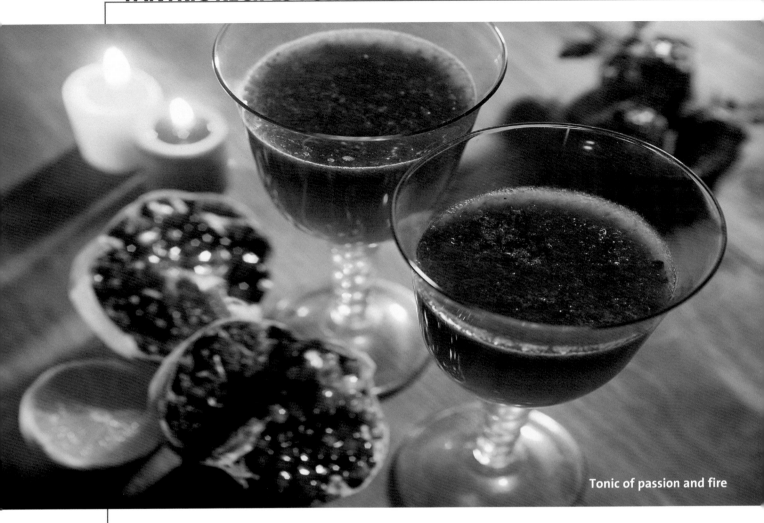

Tonic of passion and fire

Here are some recipes that will stimulate your body and increase the energetic level of your chakras. They are dishes with aphrodisiac condiments that can intensify your inner vigor and sexual energy.

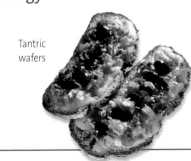

Tantric wafers

TANTRIC WAFERS

*4 slices of whole grain bread • 3 tomatoes
2 cloves of garlic • Mozzarella
Olive oil • Black olives
Fresh basil*

1. Peel three tomatoes, cut into cubes, and mix in a bowl with chopped garlic. Add salt and pepper to taste and several leaves of basil.
2. Toast four slices of bread with a dash of olive oil and a slice of mozzarella cheese.
3. Remove bread from toaster when the cheese is melted and top generously with tomato mixture.
4. Decorate with black olives and accompany with red wine.

EGGPLANT PATE

*2 large eggplants • 1 clove of garlic
Half an onion • 2 tablespoons of plain yogurt
Olive oil • Tabasco
Salt and pepper • Cayenne pepper • Mint*

1. Wash two large eggplants, pierce with a fork, and roast in the oven until tender.
2. Let cool, then peel and combine the pulp, garlic, onion, yogurt, a dash of olive oil, a few drops of Tabasco, and salt and pepper in a food processor.
3. Put in a serving dish and decorate with a sprinkle of cayenne pepper and a mint leaf.
4. Serve the pâté with toasted bread, cheese sticks, or fresh vegetables.

APHRODISIAC SALAD

2 oz (50 g) celery • 2 oz (50 g) walnuts
10 oz (300 g) prawns • 1 can of palm hearts
3 slices of pineapple

For the dressing
1/2 cup of cream cheese • Olive oil
Salt • White pepper • Lemon juice

1. Chop the celery and nuts.
2. In a bowl, prepare a salad of prawns (cooked and peeled), palm hearts cut into slices, the chopped celery and nuts, and the pineapple cubed.
3. Prepare a dressing with the cream cheese, olive oil, salt, pepper, and lemon juice.
4. Mix dressing into the salad.

RICE WITH NUTS

5 oz (150 g) brown rice • Olive oil • Turmeric
Almonds • Walnuts
Pine nuts • Raisins
Sunflower seeds • Grated coconut
Soy sauce

1. Boil rice.
2. Meanwhile, in a frying pan or earthenware pot, mix olive oil, turmeric, ginger, pepper, almonds, walnuts, pine nuts, raisins, sunflower seeds, and coconut. Sautee together for five minutes.
3. Add to the rice and serve with a few drops of soy sauce.

VEGETABLE CURRY

2 oz (50 g) green beans • 2 oz (50 g) broccoli
1 squash • 1 eggplant • Salt and pepper

For the sauce
1 cup coconut milk • 2 cups water • Basil
Ginger • Curry • 2 cloves garlic

1. Mix coconut milk, water, basil, ginger, garlic, and curry. Boil for about ten minutes.
2. Add sliced green beans, broccoli flowers, and cubed squash and eggplant.
3. Add salt and pepper to taste and cook on a low flame until the vegetables are done.

SEAFOOD PASTA

5 oz (150 g) whole grain spaghetti
9 oz (250 g) king prawns

For the sauce
1 onion • 1 clove of garlic
Olive oil • 1/2 cup of white wine
200 cup (200 ml) cream • Parmesan cheese
Salt and pepper • Nutmeg

1. Cook spaghetti in water with a little salt, drain.
2. In a saucepan, heat some olive oil, add onion, garlic, and peeled prawns, and cook until golden brown. Flambè with white wine until the alcohol evaporates, then add the cream. Season with salt, pepper, and nutmeg.
3. Serve spaghetti with liberal sauce and parmesan cheese.

TONIC OF FIRE AND PASSION

2 large pomegranates
1 teaspoon rose water
2 cups of ice water or sparkling wine
Lemon juice • Honey

Peel and take the seeds out of the pomegranates, and mix in a blender with the rose water, ice water or sparkling wine, lemon juice, and honey to taste.

COSMIC NECTAR

1 lb strawberries
2 cups (1/2 l) soy milk or ice water
Ginger • Orange or lemon zest
1 or 2 tablespoons honey • Cayenne pepper

Liquefy strawberries with soymilk or ice water, and add a pinch of ginger, orange, or lemon zest, and cayenne pepper, along with a few spoonfuls of honey.

FRESH APRICOT COCKTAIL

1 lb apricots without pits
3 tablespoons honey
2 tablespoons corn starch
6 cups (1 1/2 l) orange juice • 1/2 cup water
1 tablespoon plain gelatin

Decoration
Cherries or strawberries • Chopped almonds

1. Liquefy the apricots with honey, cornstarch, and orange juice.
2. Put the mixture in a saucepan and cook on low heat until it thickens, stirring continuously with a wooden spoon.
3. Heat the water and gelatin for five minutes.
4. Add to the apricot mixture and mix well.
5. Serve in glasses and garnish with red cherries or strawberries, and chopped almonds. Drink cold.

SWEET PLEASURES

5 oz (150 g) butter • 7 oz (200 g) fresh oats
7 oz (200 g) cacao • 7 oz (200 g) chopped nuts
Ω cup condensed milk • Grated coconut
Vanilla extract

1. In a saucepan, melt butter, oats, and cacao. Mix well and incorporate condensed milk and a few drops of vanilla extract. Remove from heat and add nuts.
2. Once mixed to a homogenous consistency, form into small balls and coat with grated coconut.
3. Serve cold.

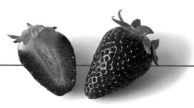

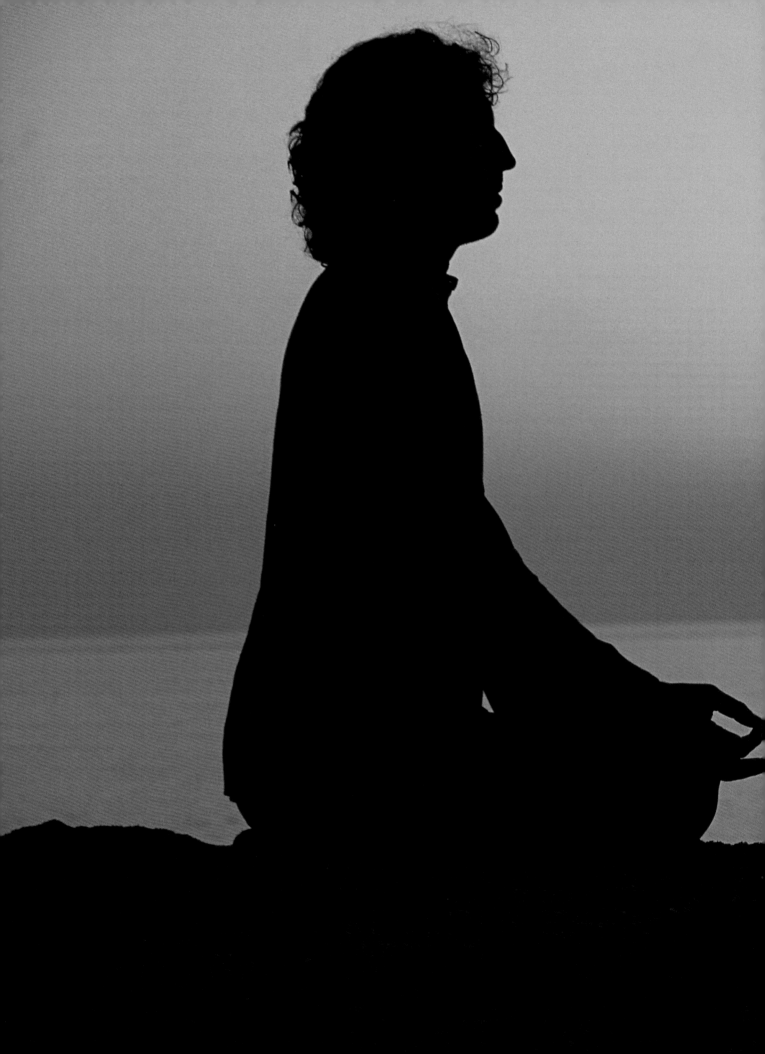

MEDITATION:
THE FIRE THAT LIGHTS THE WAY

*"Start to meditate and things will start to grow in you:
silence, serenity, happiness, sensitivity.
'Meditation' means to sink into your own immorality,
into your eternity, into your divinity."*

What Is MEDITATION?

Meditation doesn't mean centering yourself
on a certain idea, but rather ceasing the movement of the mind
to reach a state of "no mind."

Meditation is the state with which the individual centers on his or herself. It is the use of consciousness and the silence of the mind. When you practice mediation, the body achieves stillness, the nervous system is calm, and the mind ceases its constant chatter.

Although meditation lowers the number of brain waves and produces deep relaxation, its benefits are not just physical: it can also help you open deep levels of love, consciousness, peace, clarity, enthusiasm, energetic regeneration, and understanding of the mysteries of life. Tantra unites physical and spiritual healing in a holistic science.

Meditation is a "not doing," but it doesn't mean trying to do nothing in a physical sense (Tantra uses dynamic meditation and dances), but rather an attitude of disconnecting from mental work to reach the language of the soul, silence, through which you achieve expansion. Tantric meditations begin in the body in order to rid it of stress and tension, using music as a vehicle for energetic movement. After these phases, silence and stillness are natural consequences.

Meditation doesn't mean concentrating on a single point or idea (since this would imply that the mind is still "on"), but in ceasing the movement of the mind to give way to a state still unknown in the Western world, called "no mind."

THROWING THE TRASH OUT OF THE MIND, OR THE MIND OUT IN THE TRASH?

For the meditator, the mind is an impediment because it reasons, idealizes, compares, speculates, projects, believes, etc. It also thinks, for sure. Meditation is the opposite of all activity; it's neither thinking nor doing, it's Being. The being is linked to perceiving and feeling part of existence. When you are, you take consciousness that you exist; you know that you are present. Meditation heightens the inner state of perceptions.

The old quote from Hamlet, "To be or not to be, that is the question" is totally metaphysical; for Tantra it would be "To be and not to be" because in daily life you are, you control yourself as an individual, you do

MEDITATION AND ENERGY

Meditation, as a daily practice, fills closed parts of the mind and sleeping centers with vital energy. When we meditate, subtle levels of our central consciousness start to rise to the surface; the subconscious manifests. With meditation we can awaken and elevate the spiritual energy of the kundalini. This life energy nourishes, like alchemical fuel, all of the chakras and begins to develop and stimulate the individual, granting him or her spiritual abilities (ojas shakti) previously unknown.

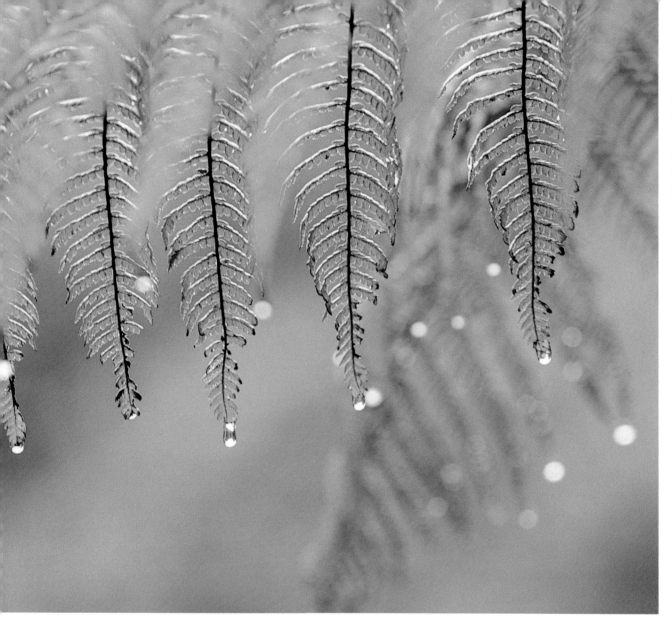

105

> **Meditation is also the falling of false masks that we use so frequently, the return to innocence and spontaneity.**

things, you move and exercise totally consciously, but you can also feel the state of not being, the vacuum, the absence of ego. Lao Tse talks about the not being, about the emptiness that fills everything; Osho developed techniques to enter the state of no mind, and meditation submerges you in the depths of yourself so you perceive the not being. An example would be a room; the walls are useful because they protect from the wind and cold, but what's really important and useful is the space inside. The walls give a shape to the space; one without the other would be impossible.

Tantra has special meditations for all types of people. Farther on I will give you a list of practices so you can tune into your own meditation.

Meditation is a state, not an activity. To meditate means being without inner conflicts or insecurities, perceiving the constant presence of our inner center. It is the encounter with the divine essence that does not belong to any organization nor has a name; the supreme power in the life of a human being, freedom.

When you enter a state of meditation you will feel freedom. And meditating every day, you drink from the fountain of your own soul so your personality aligns with your being.

Meditation is also the falling of false masks that we use so frequently, the return to innocence and spontaneity. Normally, people act on instinctive impulse from the lower chakras, or from habit or interest of the ego. Meditation, on the other hand, is feeling and acting from the deepest space of the heart and soul.

WITHOUT EMOTION AND WITHOUT MIND

In order to elevate the kundalini through meditation, you must first purify the body emotionally and mentally. Daily practice, emotional unblocking, and purification and silencing of the mind are all necessary to elevate the vital power of the fire of the spirit. If a novice needs to work on meditation to strengthen himself first, the ascent of the kundalini will come sooner or later.

An emotion is a movement of energy from inside outward, and if an individual represses or doesn't assimilate emotions, they will need to experience a catharsis to free themselves from this mental and emotional weight. Only then will they eliminate the inner blockages that impede the evolution of the soul.

When the emotional body is blocked and the energetic flow obstructed, it is like a short circuit. Mediation purifies the emotions and the mind, one through the flourishing of expression, and the other through silence.

INNER SPACE

Thanks to internal cleaning we can sink into our interior and be renewed, with an inner space of calm, happiness, and lucidity. When this space emerges, we feel the connection with the universe—that "we are like the sky, without limits."

This sacred space of light, consciousness, and ecstasy is the fruit of meditation. Bringing it into daily life is a tantric art that we must learn, without thoughts or worries.

Upon entering the world of Tantra, we are artists of the spirit, of our own lives, and happiness will be the consequence of writing our script with an open, meditative consciousness.

The tantric space gives birth to celebration, to love, and to unity of the bipolar currents inside us: both the electric and masculine, and the magnetic and feminine become one.

Deepening means finding this inner being that is love; feeling fully alert and alive, and celebrating the existence that flows through us. It is being in the exact point where magic and the miracle of being dance, and turning toward freedom where there are not chains, only wings.

SEEKING ETERNITY

We look, through different paths, for something that we can only intuit. From the brahamacharya to the drug addict, from the meditator to the gardener, we are all in pursuit of an expansion of consciousness toward divinity. Although we're like fish in the water, we're not conscious of it and so we look.

But aren't Buddha and Jesus eternal? Aren't Dali and Mozart as well? They have left us something that humanity will never forget and if we stop to think about it, we realize that the most we can do in life is artistic, and connect our souls with divinity.

Tantra insists on capturing the present. Samadhi is hidden in the corners of every soul, like a tiger ready to pounce.

Meditating is deepening the hidden tunnels of the spirit; burning layers of the subconscious and transcending the ordinary mind.

WHAT HAPPENS IN THE BRAIN

Everything that happens during meditation (whose first and foremost step is relaxation) has been subject to study, which has resulted in some revealing discoveries. Our brains produce uninterrupted electromagnetic waves at various frequencies, measurable by an electroencephalograph, that typically fall into four groups:

1. Beta waves:
From 21 to 14 cycles per second, these are present in rational, wakeful activity.

2. Alpha waves:
From 14 to 7 cycles per second, these belong to creative or imaginative activities.

3. Theta waves:
From 7 to 4 cycles per second, linked to dreams and astral journeys.

4. Delta waves:
From 4 to 1/2 cycles per second, this is the state of Samadhi, the enlightenment of the soul.
It has been observed that relaxation produces a slowing of activity in the neurons to the production of alpha waves. In a normal state of wakefulness, the waves produced by each neuron can have very different frequencies; on the other hand, in some situations (especially during mediation) the brain waves produced by each neuron tend to be more synchronized on the same frequency. Thus it creates a single harmonized wave; and synchronization that resumes a meditative state and represents the state of mystical unity with All. Meditation induces the production of serotonin and endorphins in the brain. The first is a hormone that helps with relaxation and facilitates sleep, while endorphins are called "happiness hormones": analgesics produced naturally in the organism that provide wellbeing and completeness.

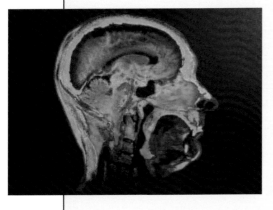

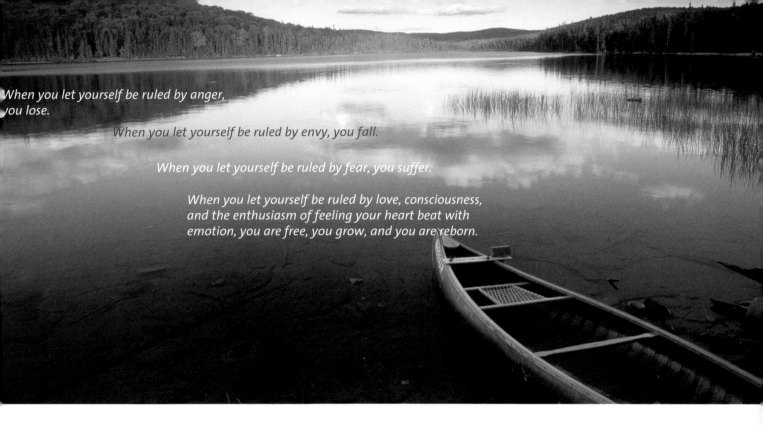

When you let yourself be ruled by anger, you lose.

When you let yourself be ruled by envy, you fall.

When you let yourself be ruled by fear, you suffer.

When you let yourself be ruled by love, consciousness, and the enthusiasm of feeling your heart beat with emotion, you are free, you grow, and you are reborn.

When we wake up every morning, we have the possibility to take new paths, to live a new day. Eternity is waiting for us, and when we detach from space and time we flow with this eternal consciousness. This is why Tantra emphasizes sex: in sex we transcend time, something that can also happen with laughter, painting, meditation, cooking, or biking. Everything can serve as the moment of inner light, when love and the present collide within you.

All of the wise men of the past have said: "Being conscious must be a habit twenty-four hours a day." When we live in the mind, most of the time it plays tricks that prevent us from enjoying the marvelous space that already exists inside us and which we can enter just by changing our state: eternity.

You have to realize that every second is vital. In each breath there is the possibility of crossing the inner bridge, so we need to throw out worries and controls and set out to live what really makes sense, realizing that eternity is present in a hug, a look, a bird on a branch. Calm breathing,

LETTING GO

If we observe life we see that many things happen because there is no resistance—they adapt to flow constantly. The eagle lets itself be carried by the wind; the boat, by the currents; and the fire, by the air. There are so many things that let themselves be carried by something unseen.

Why do human beings let things carry them away? Anger, envy, and fear, for example.

When you let yourself be ruled by anger, you lose.
When you let yourself be ruled by envy, you fall.
When you let yourself be ruled by fear, you suffer.
When you let yourself be ruled by love, consciousness, and the enthusiasm of feeling your heart beat with emotion, you are free, you grow, and you are reborn.

You can't allow anyone to block your flow through life; your will to let yourself be taken by what you feel; your desire for freedom. Letting yourself go implies risk, adventure, emotional riches, and takes us from the languishing river of routine into the ocean, to the expansion of the soul, a development that we crave from the deepest part of our being.

Close your eyes and breathe deeply and let yourself be carried back to your home: your heart, the beating of love, the inner flight to freedom.

a silent mind, and an open soul are guides in the darkness that intuitively guide us to the eternal.

This search is an individual game that will become collective when the last of the living beings cross the threshold from subconscious to the Supreme Consciousness.

When two beings share a tantric love, it is no longer a woman who loves a man, a mother who loves a son, or a grandson who loves a grandmother, but only a soul loving the energy that the other transmits, whoever it is, and is ultimately God loving himself.

TANTRIC SADHANA

Spiritual training

Sadhana, the fundamental pillar of Tantra, should be practiced daily in order to achieve results. Whether it is individual or in partners, it will noticeably increase your level of energy, connection to life, and inner clarity. Choose exercises and meditations most tuned in to the life stage you are going through. Remember some principles:

1. Take sadhana like a conscious game, not an obligation. Enjoy it.
2. Don't over do it with exercises, but don't put it off either.
3. Always let yourself be guided by the rhythm of your breathing: it should match your consciousness.
4. Don't worry about the results, these will come naturally.
5. Write down in a notebook each new sensation, state of consciousness, or symptom of the movement of the kundalini. Don't worry if you feel strong or low emotions; you are cleansing yourself in a period of catharsis.
6. You can combine some exercises to choose which one to work on, or dedicate yourself to experimenting with a specific one.
7. Respect your body like a temple; your sadhana, like a creative work; and yourself like a being of light who is returning home.

108

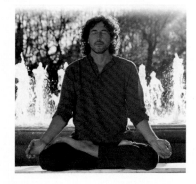

PURIFICATION OF THE BODY

EXERCISE 1

▼ Sattvic foods: fruits, vegetables, pastas, grains, nuts, fish, etc.
▼ Deep, conscious breathing
▼ Dances and yoga to move energy
▼ Oil the body and give self-massages to eliminate tension and blockages in repressed areas.

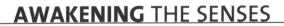

AWAKENING THE SENSES

EXERCISE 2

▼ See the beauty in all parts of life
▼ Smell the perfumes of nature
▼ Touch objects, feel through touching
▼ Hear the subtlest sounds
▼ Enjoy food

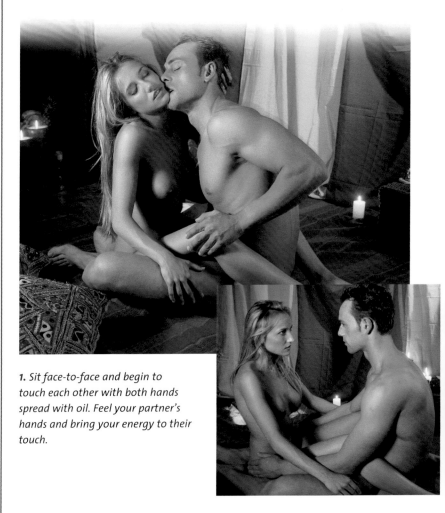

1. Sit face-to-face and begin to touch each other with both hands spread with oil. Feel your partner's hands and bring your energy to their touch.

2. Look each other in the eyes, intensifying the sense of sight. After five minutes, close your eyes and bring your energy to your ears, coming together to hear the other's breathing.

CONNECTING WITH THE ELEMENTS

▼ *Watch a fire dance, feel its heat*
▼ *Breathe the fresh air*
▼ *Touch and smell the earth*
▼ *Ritual bathing in water*

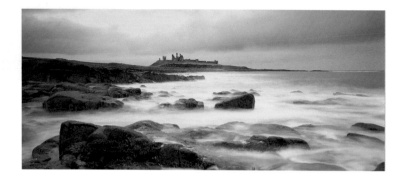

CLEANSING AND SILENCING THE MIND

▼ *Observe your thoughts without identifying with them*
▼ *Empty the mind with gibberish (sounds without logic or intellect, like those of a child or speaking an unknown language)*
▼ *Move the energy from the lower chakras to the upper ones with deep breaths*

ELMINATING NEGATIVE EMOTIONS

▼ *Fear of the future, taking consciousness of what is real*
▼ *Anger and disputes with catharsis*
▼ *Laziness, depression, and disinterest with dynamic activity*
▼ *Criticism of others with your own creativity*
▼ *Don't get stuck in memories of the past*

3. The next sense to stimulate is the sense of smell, sensing your partner's personal smell, and finally, feeling their skin with your mouth, stimulating the sense of taste with a kiss or some food.

The senses open
like windows, so
the light of the
being shines out.

INTENSIFYING POSITIVE ATTITUDES TOWARD LIFE

EXERCISE 6

▼ Cultivate a daily meditation routine
▼ Live in the present, don't plan too much. Adapt to the Tao.
▼ Assimilate the teachings as you experience them
▼ Be positive
▼ Care for your vibration with exercises, attitude, company, and thoughts
▼ Enjoy everything intensely

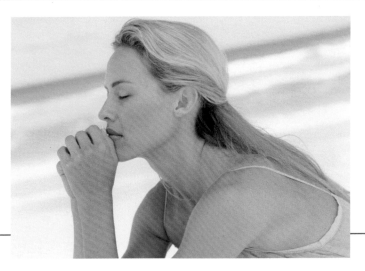

EXCHANGE OF FOOT MASSAGES

EXERCISE 7

Put oil on each other's left feet and massage gently with both thumbs for about fifteen minutes. Then do the same with the right feet. This mutual massage allows you to feel pleasure and relax at the same time. Afterward, lay face up and relax.

110

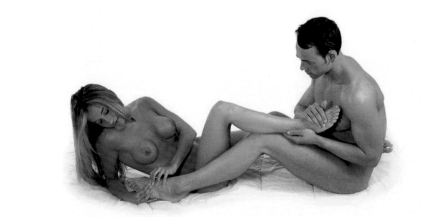

HEART CONNECTION

EXERCISE 8

Seated face-to-face, inhale deeply and slowly through the nose and exhale through the mouth, with your right hand on your partner's chest and your left hand holding theirs. The best position is the diamond pose (seated on your heels with the legs folded), although you can also do it in lotus or half lotus.

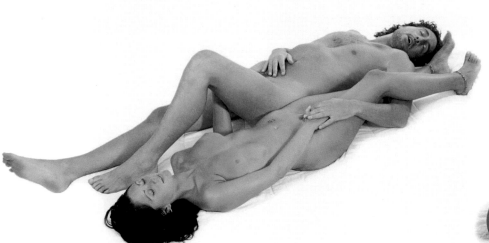

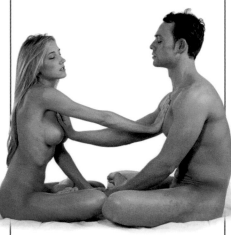

HEALING THE CHAKRAS

EXERCISE 9

Put oil on your partner's back and massage in circles, clockwise to simulate the chakras and then counterclockwise to soothe them. Start at the first chakra, in the sacral area, and work up to the head. Then repeat with your partner face up. This exercise should be accompanied by circular breathing, inhaling through the nose and exhaling through the mouth.

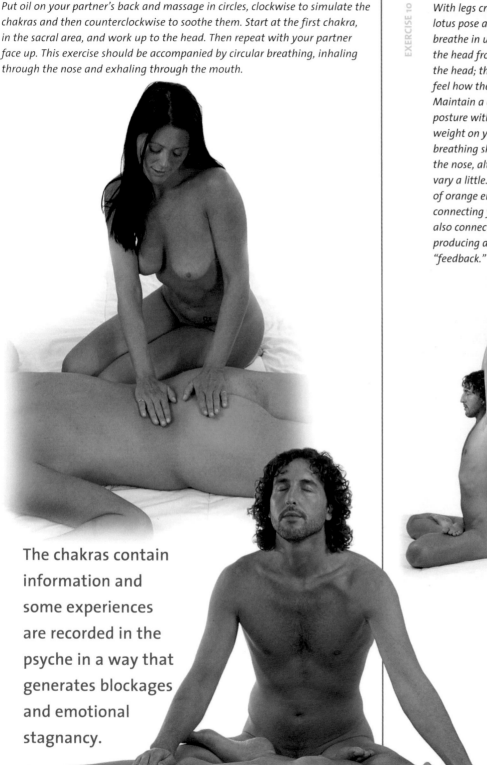

The chakras contain information and some experiences are recorded in the psyche in a way that generates blockages and emotional stagnancy.

ELEVATING THE KUNDALINI

EXERCISE 10

With legs crossed in the half lotus pose and backs together, breathe in unison, elevating the head from the sacrum to the head; this way you will feel how the energy rises. Maintain a comfortable posture without leaning your weight on your partner. Your breathing should be through the nose, although you can vary a little. Visualize a cone of orange energy rising. By connecting your backs, you also connect the chakras, producing an energetic "feedback."

111

THE COSMIC EIGHT

EXERCISE 11

Sit in half lotus and take each other's hands, crossing them: the right hand, on top, gives, and the left hand, below, receives. Forming an eight, the eternal symbol, breathe and feel the energy generated and the deep sense of unity. Breathe through the mouth.

Meditations

in pairs are authentic

orgasmic experiences.

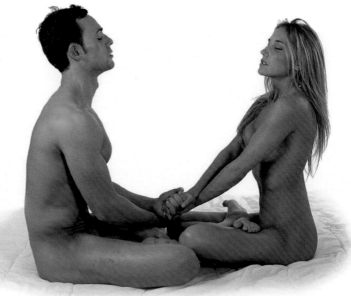

THE BOAT OF LOVE

EXERCISE 12

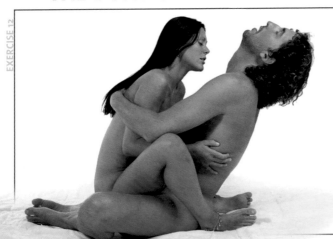

Sit in the pose of Shiva and Shakti (the man with his legs crossed and the woman with her legs open around him), embrace each other and rock forward and back. When you go backward, inhale through the mouth, and when you go forward exhale also through the mouth. Set your own rhythm, until it starts to slow a little. This important exercise can bring you both to orgasm within a few minutes through intense breathing.

THE WAVE

EXERCISE 13

Standing with feet shoulder width apart and knees slightly flexed, bring your hands and head toward the ground, inhaling deeply through the nose. Then carry your torso up fluidly, like a wave of energy, opening your arms to the side of your chest as you exhale through the mouth with a robust "aaahhhh . . ."

Don't let your head or neck stay rigid, your whole body should move dynamically and flexibly. Repeat ten to twelve times.

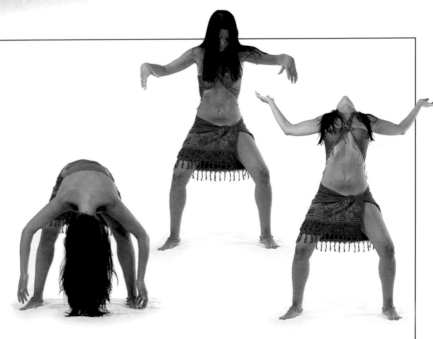

HEALING THE CHAKRAS

The consciousness of a person can be stuck in one chakra, and this means the kundalini can't rise. Every blockage of energy generates pain in the physical body; sometimes your chest or head hurts, others have a knot in their throat. The chakras need care and attention; just as computer disks contain data, the chakras hold information about the human being in their different ways of focusing on life, their desires, or their particular characteristics. To start, one partner lies face down and the other begins the healing. The exercise consists of laying two hands on each chakra for three minutes, visualizing how the energy penetrates your head, through your hands, and into your partner's chakra. Add an affirmation that gradually eliminates concepts, beliefs, and blockages that exist. When hands are on the chakras, both should practice circular breathing, inhaling through the nose and exhaling through the mouth.

Duration: 20 to 50 minutes, you can do three sets.

The chakras can have the following types of blockages.

1. Muladhara Chakra
Sexual tension

2. Swadhistana Chakra
Fear of death

3. Manipura Chakra
Accumulated negative emotions (fear, anger, anguish, worry, anxiety, or low self-esteem)

4. Anahatta Chakra
Doubt, lack of confidence, inability to love

5. Vishudda Chakra
Copying and criticizing others

6. Ajna Chakra
Internal disarray, unbalanced thoughts

7. Sahasrara Chakra
Too much ego

Repeat these affirmations out loud to heal each of the chakras, from first to seventh:

1. I relax the genital area.

2. I feel the vitality in my sexual area. I am a dynamo with endless energy.

3. My solar plexus is luminous; I see a Sun that radiates power and confidence in me.

4. Like the doors of a temple, my chest opens.

5. My throat has creative energy to express.

6. Like the center of a wheel, my being is in balance while life moves around it.

7. My head delights in an infinite ocean, in which I am pure consciousness and joy. The death of the ego is the birth of the soul.

Enjoy!

AWAKENING YOUR SEXUAL ENERGY

Lie down naked with your partner. Shakti touches Shiva's lingam and then Shiva touches Shakti's yoni. Both should breathe softly and deeply, elevating your energy while visualizing a tube of orange light that rises along the spin, from the sacrum to the brahamaranda.

By touching each other's genitals and getting excited, the kundalini awakens and begins its ascent, growing stronger with the vitality of each chakra. Don't let climax make you lose consciousness; enjoy the energy once it is awake and caress your lover's body with softness and devotion. Breathing is the key to success in the tantric formula of energy-consciousness.

When finished, breathe and transmute energy, or prepare yourselves for maithuna.

Duration: 15 to 20 minutes.

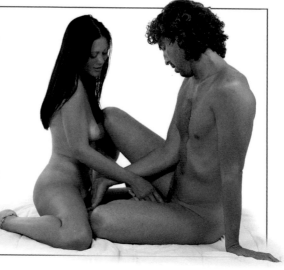

113

STRENGTHENING THE PC MUSCLE

EXERCISE 17

Also called the muscle of love, the pubococcygeus muscle is found at the midpoint between the pubis and coccyx. With the control of this important muscle, a man can control his ejaculation, and a woman can be multi-orgasmic. Lie face down and contract and relax this muscle for five minutes, at least in the morning and afternoon. When urinating, you can also contract and relax the PC muscle for three to five seconds, stopping and starting the stream of urine.

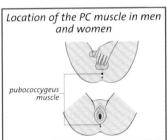

Location of the PC muscle in men and women

pubococcygeus muscle

THE GREAT SPIRAL

EXERCISE 18

Sitting with back straight, legs crossed, and hands palm up on your knees, touch thumbs to index fingers; this means that the individual soul unites with the universal soul, creating a circle. Visualize a motor of energy in the sacral region: the kundalini rising, chakra by chakra, in the form of a violet and orange spiral. Let the energy rise through deep breathing until you feel the immensity of consciousness when it reaches the seventh chakra. Meditate a few minutes on the high and let the fresh feeling of expansiveness radiate from the top of your head, like rain that nourishes the cells of the consciousness.

THE THIRTY-SIX TATWAS

EXERCISE 16 (advanced)

This exercise in attitude and consciousness is done little by little and incorporated into daily life.

Elements:
11. Earth: touch it and feel it
2. Water: bathe yourself ritually
3. Air: hold your breath a few seconds then breathe deeply
4. Fire: dance around it or meditate in silence, observing the flames

Senses:
5. Smell: appreciate smells
6. Taste: sample flavors

7. Form: observe your naked body in the mirror
8. Touch: touch something or someone
9. Sound: repeat the OM, the mantra of the mantras

Organs of action:
10. Feet: walk meditatively, massaging them
11. Word: speak, sing, communicate
12. Hand: creative capacity
13. Anus: evacuate with consciousness of the body's movement, absorb and eliminate
14. Sex: intermittent urination and conscious sexual function

Organs of perception:
15. Skin: feel it, moisturize it, mobilize energy
16. Eyes: walk with eyes closed, feel what happens inside

17. Tongue: enjoy foods
18. Nose: smell something, breathe
19. Ears: hear the subtlest sounds

Mind:
20. Mind: observe your thoughts a while, take note of them and their source
21. Intelligence: develop an idea from a new and innovate perspective
22. Objective ego: eliminate the false idea that "I" do something and feel how you are an instrument of the divine
23. Prakriti: material, related to Shakti: the feminine power, receptiveness
24. Purusha: spirit, related to the lingam: principle that penetrates the material, weaving events

114

THE MAGIC MIRROR

EXERCISE 19

Sit in front of a mirror and observe your image with total detachment. Observe your face and body, then look directly into your eyes; until they fill with tears. This contemplation awakens the deep consciousness of energy and detachment from the physical body. Tantra says that with this exercise, it's possible to see the face we had in a past life. Don't use a broken mirror.

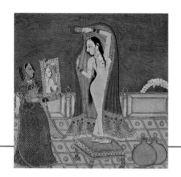

OBSERVING THE FLAME OF A CANDLE

EXERCISE 20

Place a lit candle in front of you and sit in lotus or half lotus, concentrating all your eyes' energy in the dancing of the flame. Do this for ten minutes then close your eyes; you will see the flame with your eyes closed. Fix this image in your mind.

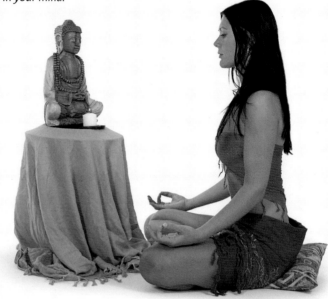

Shields to perceive totality:

25. Time: tear down the illusion of time, feel the eternal

26. Space: tear down the illusion of limited space, awaken omnipresence

27. Deficiency: eliminate the belief that we are not perfect

28. Limitation of knowledge: awaken intuitive knowledge (prajna)

29. Creativity: don't limit creativity, use it to do something productive

30. Global illusion: believe that something is real when it is an illusion

Deep perception of the whole:

31. Take consciousness of your own nature: meditate in silence on a pure state of origin

32. Subjectivity granted by power: feel your inner power

33. Universal I: the center of the universe is inside us, the essence, the soul

34. Shakti: the goddess, the feminine, in your body and in your surroundings

35. Shiva: the god, the masculine, in your body and in your surroundings

36. Complete fusion of the two into One

The kundalini, stimulated in many ways, will rise in a spiral of energy.

115

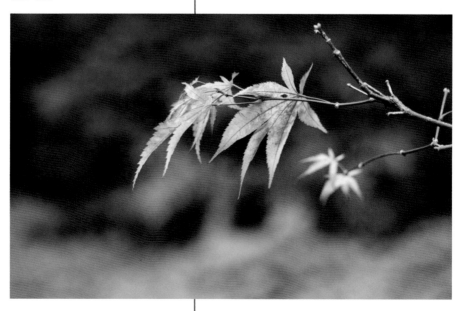

TANTRA BEFORE MAKING LOVE

This meditation is to be done before maithuna.

Prepare the setting with cushions, candles and incense, a basket of fruit and drinks. Take each other's hands, sit face-to-face, and awaken the senses: first, sight, looking at your partner's body with total devotion; then, with eyes closed, emit sounds through exhalation to increase the eroticism and sensuality; smell your partner's perfumed skin; stimulate taste by kissing their body softly and meditatively; and finally, run your hands over their body, activating touch and the language of the skin. After awakening the senses, breathe through your mouth slowly and deeply for five minutes. This will increase consciousness and energy even more.

Softly and deeply, inhale three times and hold the air for three seconds in each chakra, until it reaches the seventh. Visualize the whole lineage of tantric masters, full of light, protected, and elevating the kundalini of sex to the spirit along the astral column.

Now you are ready to live Tantra and feel the eternity through sexual ritual.

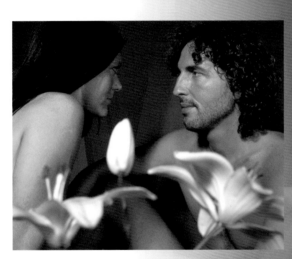

CREATING THE CIRCLE OF LOVE

Sit naked, face-to-face, look each other in the eyes, and hold hands for about five minutes. Then, close your eyes and breathe in unison. Your breathing should be deep and circular, without space in between. Thanks to this respiratory circuit, soon you will have the sensation of forming a circle with both energies, which allows the detachment from the individual ego and the sensation that both of you fuse with the cosmos through the other.

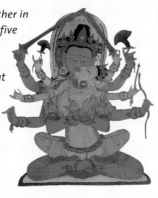

WHERE ARE YOU?

Too young
to meditate.

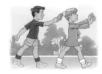

Too active
to meditate.

Too impulsive
to meditate.

Too in love
to meditate.

Too busy
to meditate.

Too tired
to meditate.

Too worried
to meditate.

Too old
to meditate.

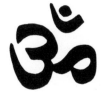

Too late
to meditate.

Such is life.

EXERCISE 23

THE MAGIC SOUND

For Tantra, the repetition of a mantra is a science. OM, the sound of the universe, can be used by couples to mix and fuse their energies. Do it daily for a few minutes, or before making love. The OM attracts positive energies from all existence, although you can also use specific mantras for each ritual.

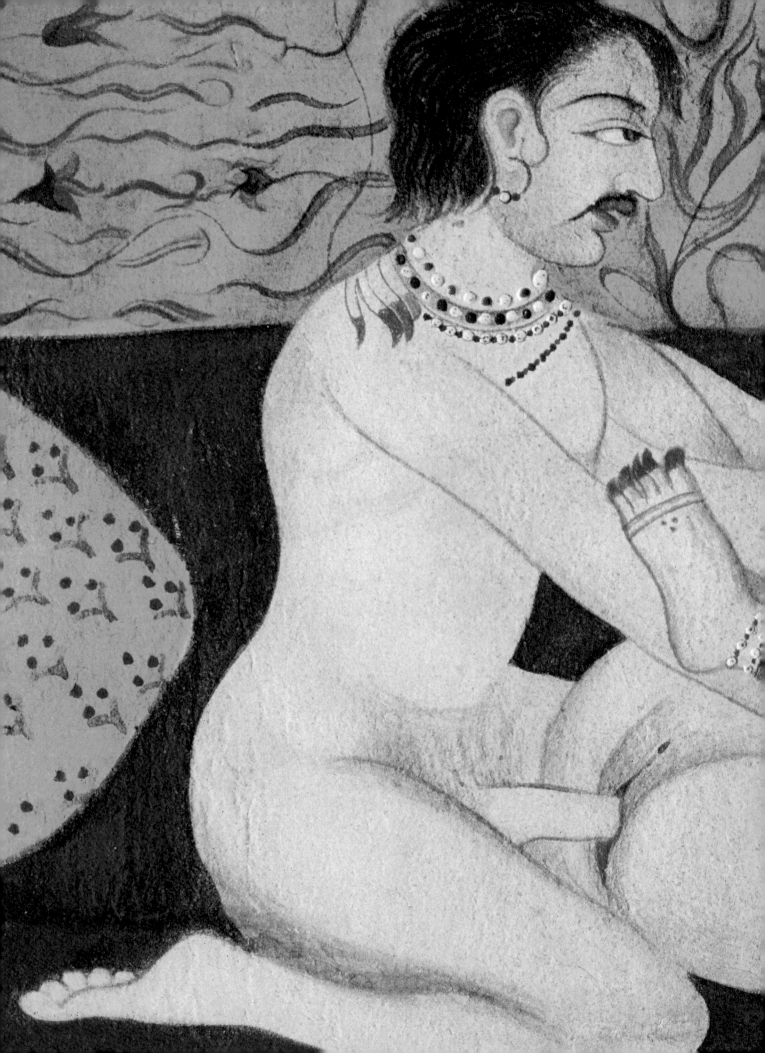

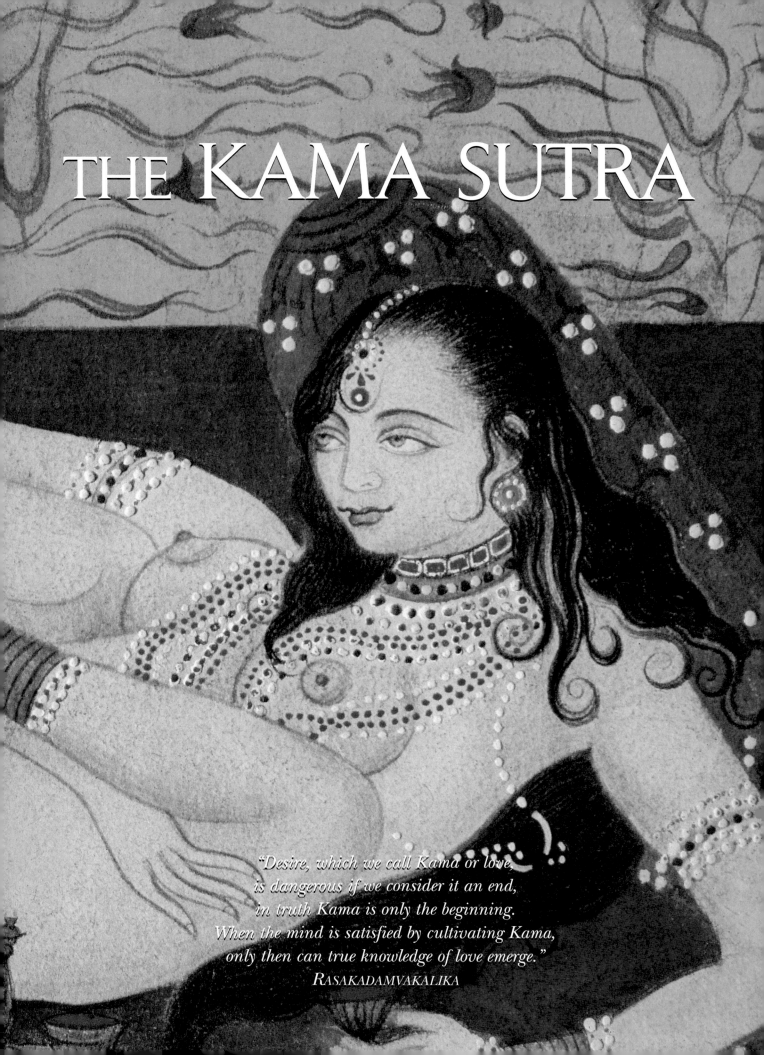

THE KAMA SUTRA

*"Desire, which we call Kama or love,
is dangerous if we consider it an end,
in truth Kama is only the beginning.
When the mind is satisfied by cultivating Kama,
only then can true knowledge of love emerge."*
RASAKADAMVAKALIKA

The Wisdom OF DESIRE

If sexual desire is repressed it can become an obsession;
from there the necessity to satisfy it in order to transcend it.
In this sense, the Kama Sutra offers Tantra the tools to overcome
all types of repressions and taboos.

Kama Sutra is a lovely word formed by "kama" ("desire") and "sutra" ("wisdom"), and the name of an ancient Indian document that, as the name indicates, intelligently explains the wisdom of human desire.

Although the Kama Sutra is not part of the body of Tantric texts, the objective of this book is to bring you closer to its concepts and practices. Written by Vatsyayana and covering human sexuality, the Kama Sutra reflects extensively on all the corners of sexual life and its secrets; above all, concerning the increase of energy through special postures and knowledge of the body and its powers.

Some amazingly beautiful works of art and relief sculptures in stone (especially in the cities of Khajuraho and Konarak in India) have been made of the positions in the Kama Sutra, which reflect a golden age of pleasure, sex, and consciousness.

Unfortunately, many with closed minds have written these monuments off as pornographic, without knowing their hidden meaning; Muslim fanatics have destroyed seventy temples, leaving only about thirty remaining. The purpose of the temples was that whoever wanted to enter should first meditate in certain poses until their mind was emptied of sexuality or desire; that is to say, they must enter with a clean mind. The objective of the images therefore was to meditate on desire and sex in order to be free of it, transcend it, and reach a stage of greater energy and emptiness.

Sex is very good for Tantra, but we still seek to go farther. If one represses sex, it will always be on their mind, while if one satisfies desire they transcend it. It's like when you are hungry: you are always thinking of food, but once you've eaten and are satisfied, you don't need to think about it anymore.

Tantra alludes to beauty and nudity. A naked body is natural: animals and plants are naked, yet human beings have made nudity an enormous taboo. For example, on nudist beaches not everyone dares to be naked. So many people repress the urge, when it is so natural, free, and enjoyable to be without clothes that the body is invigorated, the cells are energized, your skin glows, and your spirit returns to its origins. Of course you can't be naked in the streets, but in your house you can do it daily. I don't understand how people can be in their house wearing clothes and shoes, since the body tires more easily this way.

It may surprise you to know that in the Victorian era, moralists covered the feet of chairs because they were considered pornographic! They also insisted on dressing their dogs when they went outside. Truly, sexual repression has generated serious pathologies.

120

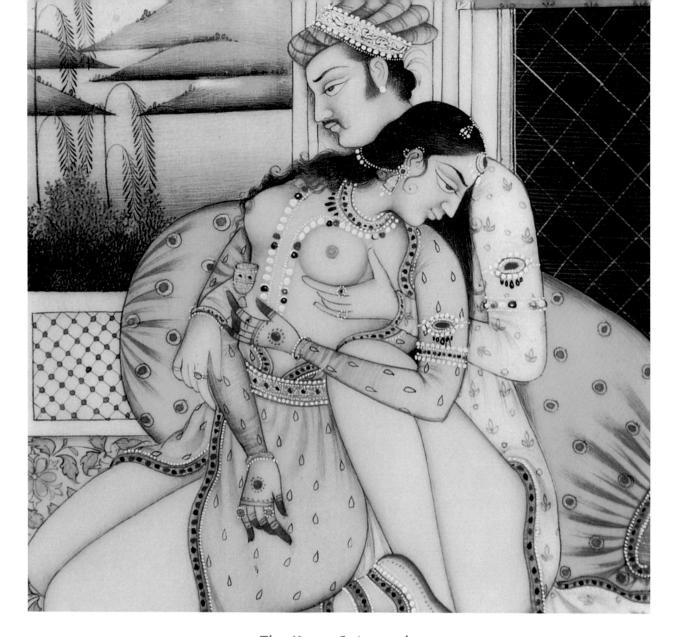

The Kama Sutra offers the tools to make the act of loving conscious, serene, and meditative; to heal the psychosexual wounds that humanity has carried on its back. Everything done in the Kama Sutra remains latent in the fantasies of the human mind, subconsciously, so desire constantly emerges because it's gone unsatisfied. And if you don't know something, you can't move past it.

OBJECTIVE

The objective of the Kama Sutra is to awaken intelligence and sexual energy, as well as to eliminate taboos built up in human nature, in order to enter an inner state of returning to innocence, naturalness, and acceptance.

The *Kama Sutra* seeks to awaken intelligence and sexual energies, thus eliminating taboos.

When you develop sexual energy and feed off of it, your internal level of creativity increases. The artists that did the sculptures based on the Kama Sutra must have had an immense energetic vibration. If you observe these sculptures with an open mind, you won't see anything perverse or por-nographic, only a reflection of what you have inside. If you are natural, you will see it as a natural act; if your mind is burdened with sex you will see your moral burden, fears, traumas, or repressions.

DO YOU MAKE LOVE OR DOES LOVE MAKE YOU?

I've come to the conclusion that we do not make love but rather love makes us, given that it makes us, molds us, and connects us. When love (not just sex) appears, it produces a transformation of consciousness, so that if we look at the deep meaning of "to make," it disappears, leaving only a state: that of being love.

And love is not simply an activity, but a state of being. One is love.

Love changes reality because it is an inner state, of consciousness filled with luminosity. It is the manifestation of divinity on Earth, of the heart that changes. You are filled with enthusiasm, vitality, and a positive outlook on life. The lens you see through becomes transparent and magnifying. Your eyes and soul fill with effervescence.

Sexual positions for entering love are the art of the Kama Sutra. Through these positions, the energy travels through your body in different ways to fill you with pleasure, satisfaction, and consciousness. And inner bliss arises when the basic desire to make love is fulfilled.

In the images of the Kama Sutra you will also find solutions for common sexual problems. Impotence, premature ejaculation, frigidness, and sexual trauma can all be healed, since the images invite experience and not the repression of desire.

DIFFERENCES BETWEEN "NATURAL" AND "OBSCENE"

There is a marked difference between what we consider natural and what can be obscene or pornographic.

You will find no trace of tension, perverseness, or anxiety in the face of a tantric individual. You will only see relaxation, peace, and contentedness. Tantra and the Kama Sutra are not the slightest bit interested in obscenity.

Tantra is the elevation of the natural to the degree of the sacred, and the sex positions of the Kama Sutra are a song of praise to free love, transcending personalities and egos. In fact, for Tantra all that is not free is not love, but control and possession.

Love is freedom, and we will find in these positions the intersection of desire and passion, meditation and consciousness united to reach the ultimate end: spiritual unity.

The obscene is found in what is degraded to the animal level. Tantra and the Kama Sutra, on the other hand, elevate the sexual so that you can feel the conscious thread that unites it with the spiritual.

I believe that you can see a clear difference between the obscene and the spiritual: one way includes heart and soul, while the other includes mind and perversion.

THE BENEFITS OF NUDITY

In Spain there are about 150 nudist beaches. Just as the Kama Sutra stimulates nudity as a natural phenomenon, nudist beaches offer the almost therapeutic opportunity to feel in harmony with Mother Nature from the most natural form we have: the body. It's very pleasant to see and feel the mood in these naturist settings: silence, pleasure, rest, and connection to the inner world. And being naked near the sea (where life originated) awakens ancestral sensations and feelings. The enormous energetic flow of nature gives all sorts of benefits to those who practice nudism:

The sun on naked skin:
▼ *Has an antiseptic effect*
▼ *Increases the vitamin D in the skin*
▼ *Helps the absorption of calcium in the bones*
▼ *Improves the immune system*
▼ *Increases the number of white blood cells in the blood and the concentration of red blood cells, which transport oxygen to the tissues*
▼ *Stimulates the hormonal system, especially the pituitary gland and thyroid*
▼ *Tones the nervous system and stimulates the psyche*
▼ *Increases intellectual activity*

Contact with the sea:
▼ *Helps the remineralization of the organism*
▼ *Stimulates the circulatory system like a massage*

The air also contributes energy in the following ways:
▼ *The ocean breeze, full of oxygen and prana (negative ions), benefits health and vitality*
▼ *Increases the absorption of yodo, fundamental for good thyroid function*
▼ *Produces more serotonin, a neurotransmitter related with relaxation and tranquility*
▼ *Finally, contact with the sand stimulates the kidneys and the chakras.*

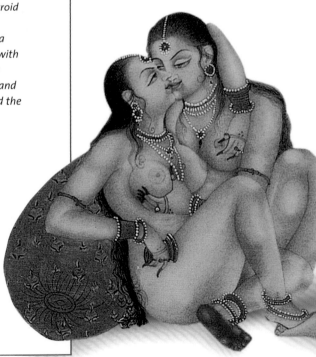

THE RITUAL BATH

Before maithuna or any energetic ritual, taking a shower is recommended. The water purifies the energetic field and predisposes the body and mind to open to the energy.

The bath is a process of purification, and cold showers have an energetic power by generating negative ions, with invigorating and regenerative properties for the body and psyche. The bath is, for Tantra, a precursor to the sexual act.

The yogic texts talk about the importance of the bath as a purifying agent, especially after a day of activity. It is best to take a bath within an hour before maithuna, since any longer you will lose the fluids and bioelectricity generated.

THE YOGA OF SLEEP

"The night of the body is the day of the soul," says a tantric proverb.

After practicing tantric love or simply going to sleep at night, Tantra recommends programming yourself to dream and remember the experiences of the astral journey. This practice is called "Yoga Nidra." For this you need to practice visualization with the mind. The dreams are not analyzed

KNOWLEDGE OF THE TANTRIC ARTS

The Kama Sutra mentions sixty-four arts and ways of applying energy. The most practical for modern men and women are:

▼ *Making perfumes*
▼ *Training the body with yoga*
▼ *Making mandalas and mystic diagrams*
▼ *Gardening and flower arranging*
▼ *Writing and composing songs and poems*
▼ *Using magic energy*
▼ *Dancing*
▼ *Preparing exotic juices and drinks*
▼ *Cooking*
▼ *Archery*
▼ *Using telepathy*
▼ *Dying your hair, painting your nails, and caring for the body*
▼ *Painting*
▼ *Solving riddles*

▼ *Reading*
▼ *Singing*
▼ *Speaking languages*
▼ *Learning dictionaries*
▼ *Getting to know a person by their particularities*
▼ *Making images in sand or working with clay*
▼ *Manual creative activities*
▼ *Sewing*
▼ *Mimicry*
▼ *Mental exercises*
▼ *Architecture*
▼ *Domestic economics*
▼ *Costumes*

like in western psychoanalysis, but rather understood by the inner master that each of us possess. There are four distinct states of consciousness: sleeping, dreaming, wakefulness, and turiya (the state of expanded consciousness).

Throughout history, many kings and emperors have counted on a team of people that dreamed to foresee the future. These visions come from a subtler world than the physical one, one you can only reach with the astral body.

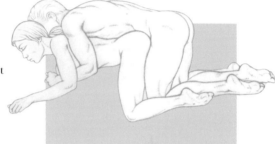

Before going to bed (after taking a bath and relaxing deeply) we practice a combined meditation and rest on our right sides. In this position, you will breathe through the left nostril, related to the right side of the brain. Stretch out your bodies and sleep together imagining that both your kundalinis connect and rise, weaving together.

It is important to go to sleep with your consciousness focused on remembering dreams. Tantra teaches that you have to concentrate in the throat chakra and visualize an OM in your center. This visualization allows you to consciously enter the world of dreams.

This initiation is a source of inspiration that will bring new ideas and feelings, more complete perceptions of existence, and the overcoming of the limits of space and time.

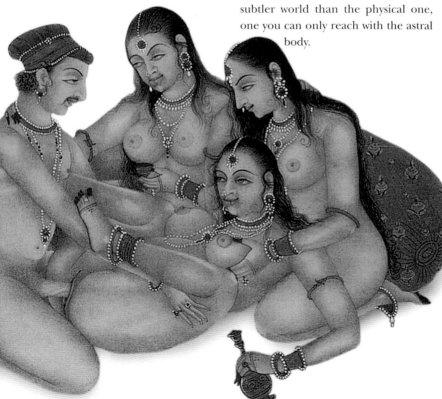

I recommend you repeat the two following tantric sutras before beginning the magic act:

1. *"Upon entering the sexual union, remain focused on the initial flame, and avoid reaching final embers."*
(FIRST SUTRA OF SHIVA WITH DEVI)

2. *"Breathing, thought, and semen are the three main elements of the potential for enlightenment. They should be harmonized and controlled consciously. The yogi that achieves unity of breathing, thought, and semen, becomes the Indestructible, gifted with transcendental spontaneity."*
(KALACHAKRA TANTRA)

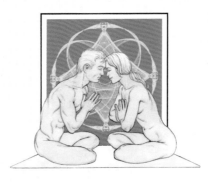

1 PARTNERS IN PRAYER

The couple meditates for a few minutes with hands at the chest in the symbol of prayer, feeling as if they are beginning a magical moment, and practice that pranayama Shiva–Shakti: when one exhales, the other inhales this air for at least seven minutes. This exchange of air and energy is the antechamber to the exchange of magic energies.

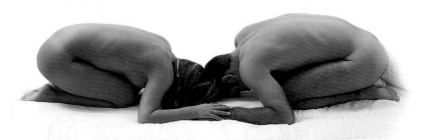

2 WORSHIPPING YOUR DIVINITY

Totally relaxed, the couple leans forward over a cushion to awaken a meditative attitude, bringing their foreheads to the ground while mentally repeating: "I worship the divinity that lives in you." Dedicate a few minutes to feeling how the mind empties of trivialities and worries to open to the supraconscious. Before beginning with the poses and penetration, it is important to practice nyasa, foreplay, stimulation of the senses, different kinds of kisses, and to enjoy food and drink.

3 THE TANTRIC EMBRACE

This position is the precursor to intimacy and penetration. The embrace is an important form of communication and connection. When the couple embraces, they overcome distance and become one. The embrace also awakens the senses of touch, smell, and taste, sensitivity, skin contact, the death of intellect, etc. It is a time when relaxation and eroticism combine, a time of devotion to the divinity that lives in your lover.

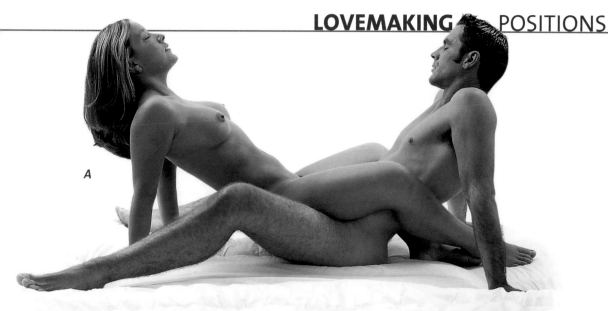

A

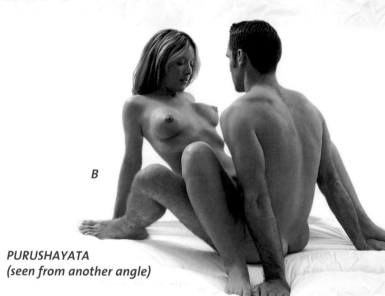

B

PURUSHAYATA
(seen from another angle)

4 PURUSHAYATA: THE WOMAN ON TOP

The man places himself with legs open, supporting himself on his arms, and the woman sits on top of him. The advantages of this position are that the Shakti initiates the movements and controls the experience. For his part, the man can relax without fear of ejaculation. It produces an important freedom for the woman that awakens her inner Shakti and the magic power she possesses. The man benefits by having his back straight so he can begin visualization and elevation of the kundalini through the chakras.

DRINKING THE NECTAR OF THE GODS

Mutual oral sex provides, in addition to pleasure and satisfaction, stimulation of the erotic organs of the body and the sharing of sacred fluids. It strengthens the sexual center of both lovers and awakens transcendental abilities. The Kama Sutra teaches us that the tongue is an important driving force that connects to sex through the central channel. When the woman is excited she transmits psychomagnetic yoni waves, which create a force field and energy that polarizes and charges in the center of the man's head. This polarizing effect causes secretions from the pineal and pituitary glands, helping both open the Third Eye. When the man is excited, he emits psychoelectric lingam waves, which help the woman elevate her kundalini in a whirlwind of ecstasy.

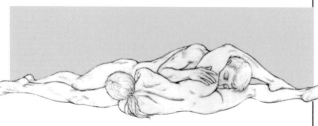

Just as a plug has two principles to generate light, the sexual game is the wise union of two poles to "turn on" the light of the soul. This sequence contains a series of asanas necessary for:

1. The balance of active and passive roles in the couple
2. The mixture of breathing poses to channel mobilized energy
3. Immobile asanas, called "poses of meditation," to activate the chakras in this moment
4. Orgasm poses

5. Attention to energetic movement
6. The transcendence of consciousness on the road to supraconsciousness
7. Rest every twenty minutes so the experiences can last three or four hours

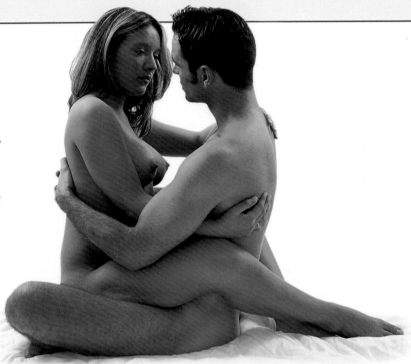

5 PURUSHAYATA in lotus

By positioning the legs in siddhasana, the lotus pose, the blood flow to the sexual area and below diminishes considerably, which allows the blood to nourish the upper body, spine, and nervous system for a moment.

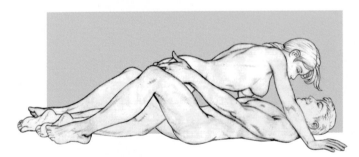

6 SHAKTI DANCES ON SHIVA

The man assumes the passive role, allowing relaxation through the Way of the Valley, and eliminating the compulsive need to ejaculate. The man becomes "feminine," associating himself with the joy of Shakti, who moves her hips in an undulating or circular motion.

The man can leave his legs open with Shakti between them, or let her open her legs for greater freedom. The man can stimulate her first chakra by introducing his ring finger a few centimeters into her anus, which will produce her first orgasms. The extremely slow movements provide pleasure that

will intensify with consciousness of the moment, the area stimulated, and the rhythm. The slow rhythm of the Way of the Valley offers you an invaluable gift: entrance to the eternity of the present. Breathing together, let the waves of pleasure and connection increase with every breath.

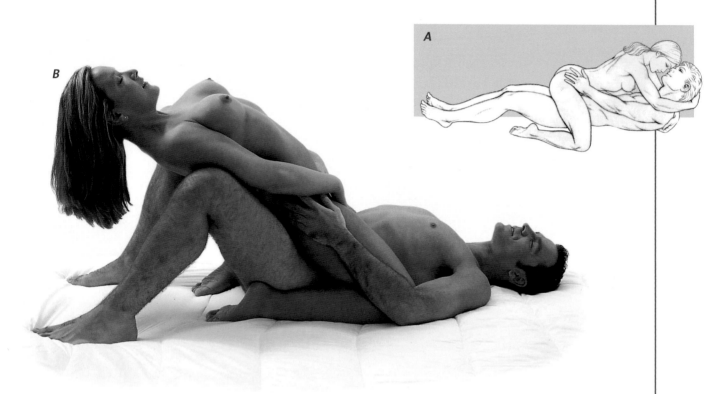

7 RAINBOW (A) AND (B)

This movement consists of two parts. The woman reclines against Shiva's folded legs (as he lies face up) and inhales slowly and deeply to open the chest and fourth chakra. When she exhales through the mouth with an "ahhhh . . ." she brings her torso to her partner's body. This interesting movement "decentralizes" attention from the genitals to let the waves of sexual energy fill the entire body. Each time Shakti goes forward, she gives her heart to Shiva and he receives it gently.

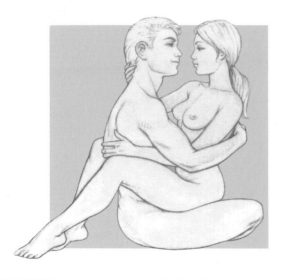

8 SUKHASANA
pose of shiva and shakti

On a carpet, with legs crossed in half lotus or lotus, the man receives his partner, who has her legs crossed. The contact goes from the gaze to the body, so this is a good asana for dedicating a few minutes to immobile meditation and breathing. You will probably feel like the "owners of the universe," full of an intense sensation of plenitude and contentedness.

127

9 VARIATION OF SUKHASANA
on a chair

For older couples or those with less flexibility, this is a good variation on the previous position, since the verticality of the spines empowers the meeting of the chakras.

10 THE DELIVERY

Shakti delivers her body in a soulful embrace. In these sacred moments, the couple reaches a deep unity, as told in the second tantric sutra: "When in such an embrace your senses feel shaken like leaves, enter this tremor."

11 ELEPHANT POSE

On foot, the woman opens her legs and lets her torso fall forward, until she touches the ground with her hands. The man, also standing, positions himself behind her and takes her hips, practicing slow and harmonious movements: circles and shakes like the steps of an elephant. It is a good position to delay or suspend ejaculation because there is no tension. When he gets close to ejaculation, the man should stop and apply different techniques:

1) Breathe intensely through the mouth for a minute or two. This locomotive breathing sends energy up, away from the genitals.
2) Apply muladhara bandha and asvini mudra.
3) Press his tongue to the roof of his mouth while raising closed eyes upward. Shakti benefits from blood flow to the brain because it nourishes the pineal gland and third eye, and facilitates new orgasms.

12 THE VINE

On foot, Shakti wraps around Shiva like a green vine on a trunk. The movements are slow, almost imperceptible. It is a moment of energetic connection as the chakras touch in the front; of union of two universal forces in the body from the contact between lingam (positive polarity) and yoni (negative polarity), and the man's nipples (negative) and woman's (positive).

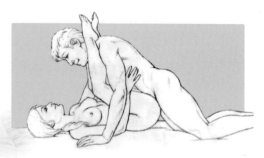

13 THE CROW

Here Shiva takes the active role, while Shakti, lying on her back, raises her legs and touches her ankles with her hands. The blood goes up, irrigating the heart and the higher chakras, and allowing pleasure to increase through deep penetration.

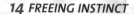

14 FREEING INSTINCT

The woman kneels with legs open and back slightly curved, and the man enters from behind, keeping his back straight. This is a position that makes it difficult to ejaculate, because the testicles are squeezed a little bit, but despite this pressure it provides a lot of pleasure and multiple orgasms. It also awakens the primal animal instinct, which should be satisfied by leaving the Way of the Valley a little to walk on the edge of the knife. It can be a position for strong, dynamic movements as much as playing with the rhythm and doing it very gently. Here breathing is vital.

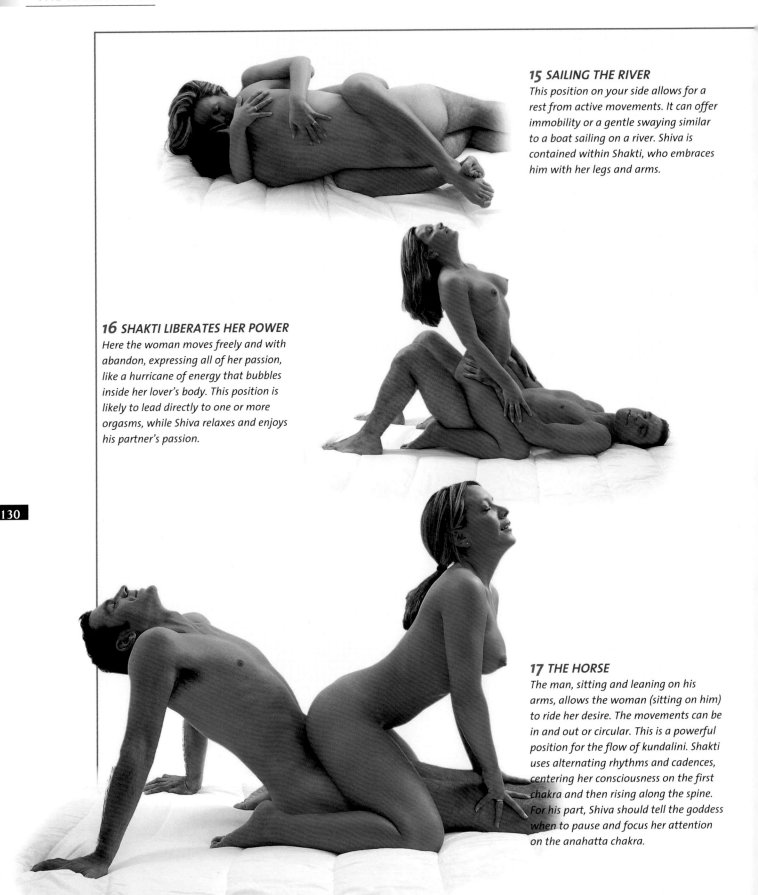

15 SAILING THE RIVER
This position on your side allows for a rest from active movements. It can offer immobility or a gentle swaying similar to a boat sailing on a river. Shiva is contained within Shakti, who embraces him with her legs and arms.

16 SHAKTI LIBERATES HER POWER
Here the woman moves freely and with abandon, expressing all of her passion, like a hurricane of energy that bubbles inside her lover's body. This position is likely to lead directly to one or more orgasms, while Shiva relaxes and enjoys his partner's passion.

17 THE HORSE
The man, sitting and leaning on his arms, allows the woman (sitting on him) to ride her desire. The movements can be in and out or circular. This is a powerful position for the flow of kundalini. Shakti uses alternating rhythms and cadences, centering her consciousness on the first chakra and then rising along the spine. For his part, Shiva should tell the goddess when to pause and focus her attention on the anahatta chakra.

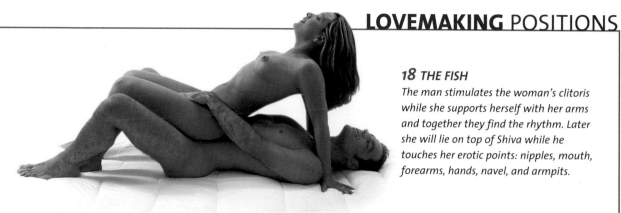

18 THE FISH

The man stimulates the woman's clitoris while she supports herself with her arms and together they find the rhythm. Later she will lie on top of Shiva while he touches her erotic points: nipples, mouth, forearms, hands, navel, and armpits.

19 THE SAILBOAT

Shakti gets on top of Shiva, looking toward his feet. The goddess' back is straight to benefit the flow of energy. She is the one who determines the rhythm of the "sailing." She can also stimulate her clitoris or touch the union of both genitals, or massage and gently pull down on Shiva's testicles to eliminate pre-ejaculatory tension.

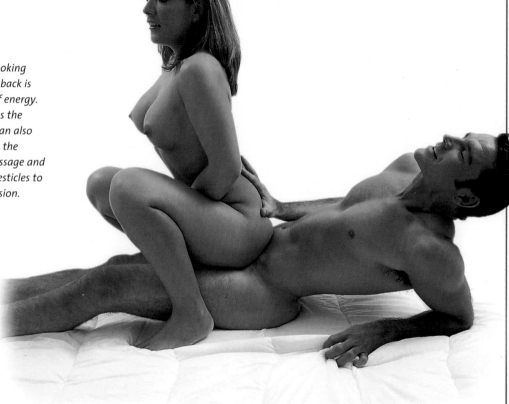

131

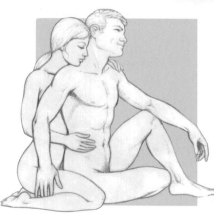

20 THE MAGNET OF THE CHAKRAS

This is a meditative rest to unite the chakras and visualize their colors, feel the plexus, breathe in unison, and develop a feather-light touch all over the body.

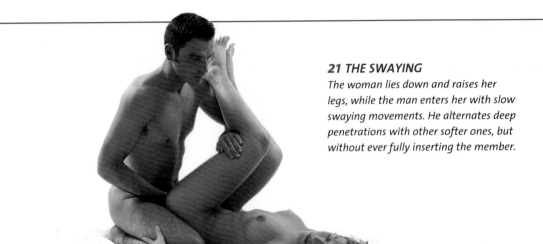

21 THE SWAYING

The woman lies down and raises her legs, while the man enters her with slow swaying movements. He alternates deep penetrations with other softer ones, but without ever fully inserting the member.

22 THE CRAB

Shiva folds his legs in diamond pose and holds Shakti's ankles. They can increase contact by looking deep into each other's eyes, which emits energy. Another variation is when Shakti folds her legs against her chest.

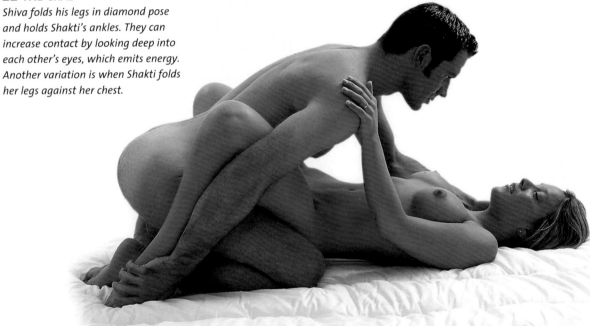

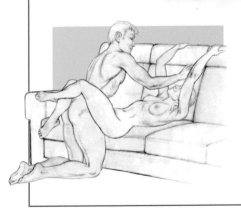

23 THE POWER OF SHIVA

Shakti lies on a chair or table and Shiva moves his pelvis as if in a dance. With strong but sensitive movements forward and back, Shiva practices the following breathing exercise: when he inserts the lingam he inhales Shakti's energy deeply, and when he takes it out, he exhales. Using a table allows Shiva to energetically and consciously develop his power. It is a great position for men with premature ejaculation, since it allows him to control the rhythm of the experience.

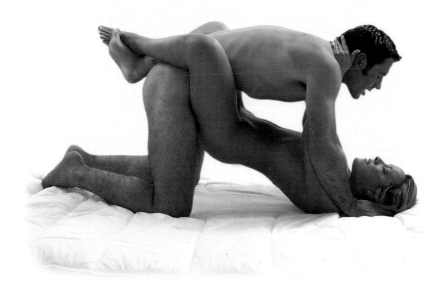

24 THE FLIGHT OF THE EAGLE

The man positions himself over the woman, who lies on her back with her legs wrapped around her partner. This is a position that allows for deep penetration and friction between their pubic hair, which activates more orgasms in Shakti.

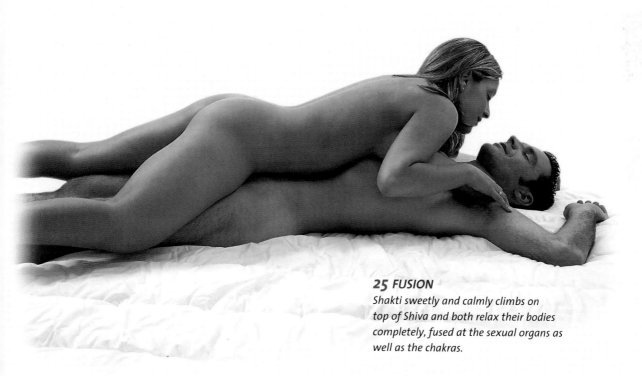

25 FUSION

Shakti sweetly and calmly climbs on top of Shiva and both relax their bodies completely, fused at the sexual organs as well as the chakras.

26 THE MOUNTAIN

Shakti is on her back with legs folded against her chest and Shiva rises like a mountain over her. This is a position for deep penetration, so the goddess should breathe intensely to prevent the energy from remaining stuck in the solar plexus and causing pain.

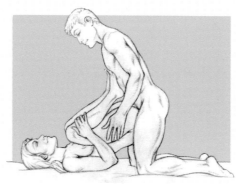

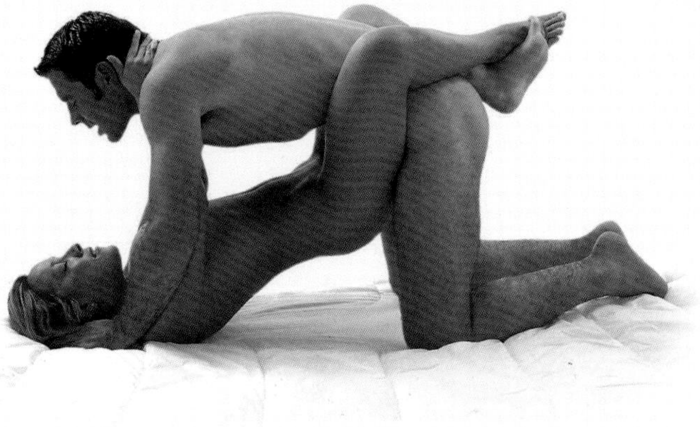

27 THE TURTLE

Shiva forms the shell and Shakti, the inside of the turtle. Embracing Shiva, with her legs behind his sacrum, the woman receives movements as slow and deep as his breathing.

28 THE SUSPENDED GODDESS

The man holds the woman, who receives energy inversely. This is good for the thyroid, pineal, and pituitary glands, and therefore the throat, forehead, and heart chakras. The blood increases its flow and circulation, and the mind enters in silence and trance. Shakti rejuvenates completely with this position.

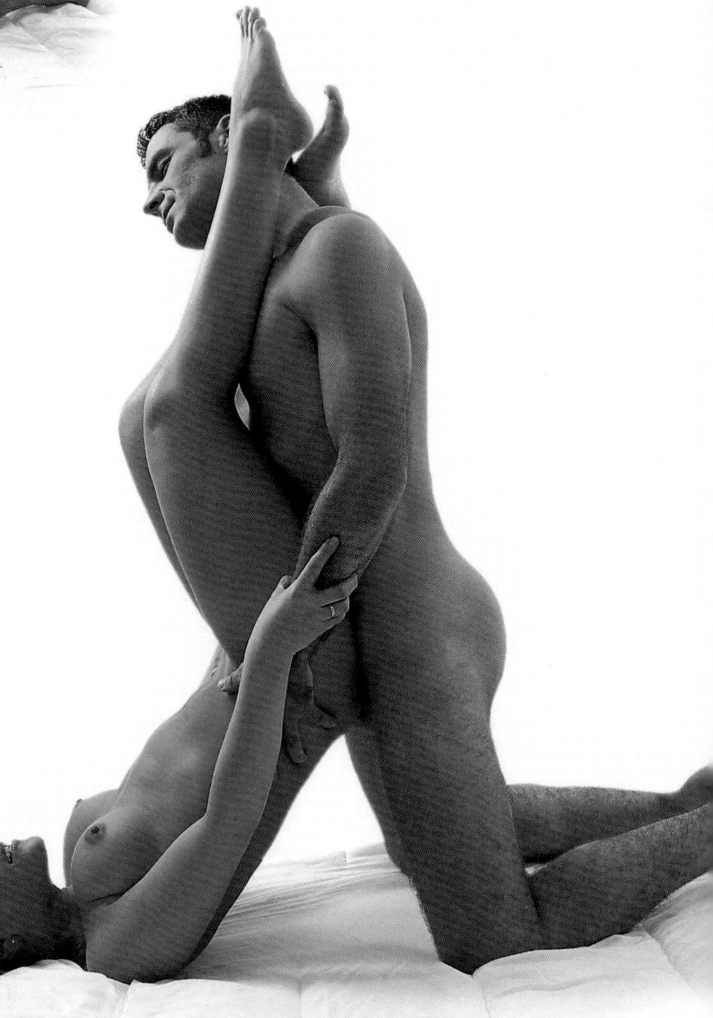

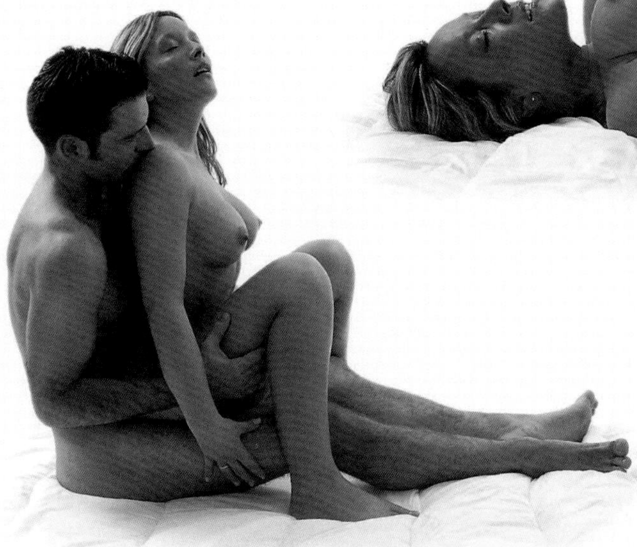

29 THE PYRAMID

The goddess positions herself on top of Shiva, with her legs open and her back to him. He holds her thighs and Shakti moves forward and back, up and down. This is a position that allows you to feel the immense heat between chest and back.

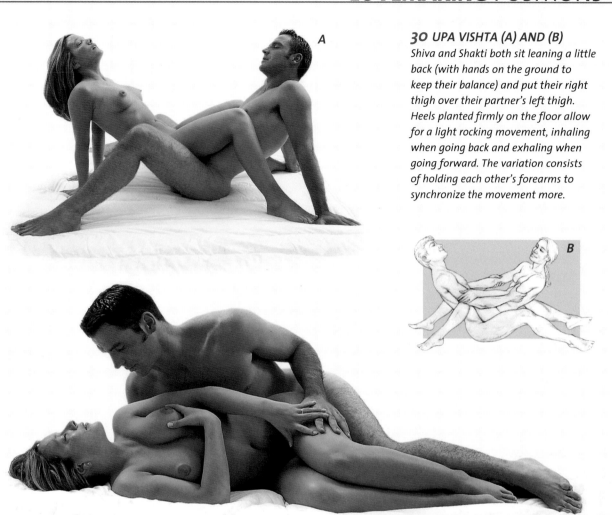

30 UPA VISHTA (A) AND (B)
Shiva and Shakti both sit leaning a little back (with hands on the ground to keep their balance) and put their right thigh over their partner's left thigh. Heels planted firmly on the floor allow for a light rocking movement, inhaling when going back and exhaling when going forward. The variation consists of holding each other's forearms to synchronize the movement more.

31 THE MOON AND THE SUN
Many mystic tantric diagrams use the colors red and white. The balance between the red and white forces of the woman and man produced during tantric sex is true energetic alchemy. They can awaken the subtle channels by visualizing the inner Sun burning in red tones (woman) and the Moon in white, refreshing tones (man) while you breathe in unison. This position also develops the psychic force between you.

32 THE OASIS OF THE GODS
This asana allows you to relax and enjoy the moment you are living. There is no penetration; only breathing, observation, and caresses.

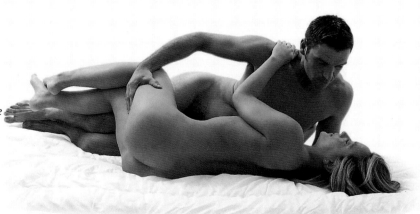

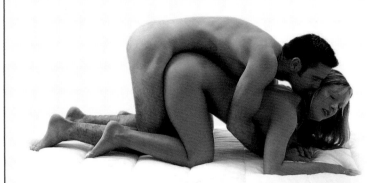

33 FINDING THE SACRED SPOT

This position gives great pleasure by intensely stimulating the G-spot. The man penetrates Shakti from behind, and she feels his lingam deeply. Given that it's difficult to maintain ejaculation, Shiva should set the rhythm.

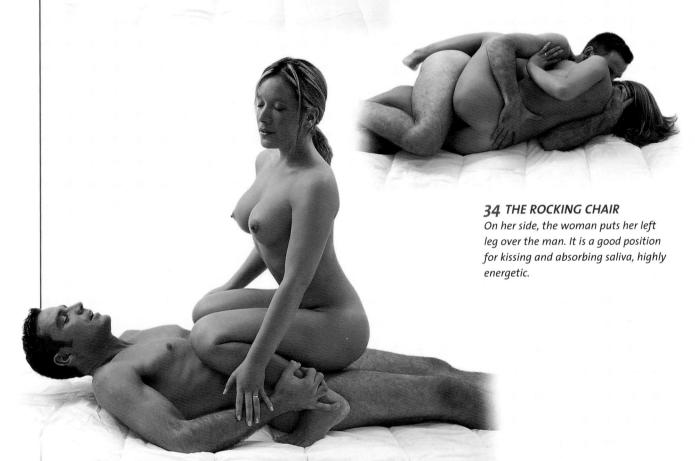

34 THE ROCKING CHAIR

On her side, the woman puts her left leg over the man. It is a good position for kissing and absorbing saliva, highly energetic.

35 THE GREAT KALI POSE

Kali is the tantric goddess of passion, transformation, and sexual pleasure. When the woman's skin and heart are full of Kali's power, she feels insatiable, gifted with great eroticism, and the desire to devour her partner. This is an asana that liberates the powerful feminine energy which the man enjoys from his passive role, becoming one with Kali. It is the moment when all repressions are vanquished and the woman is empowered. It is a naturally orgasmic position. The man breathes always slowly, deeply, and consciously, absorbing the magic energy shed by the goddess. The couple visualizes the yantra of Kali and repeats the mantra, filling their psyche with both elements. Kali can stick out her tongue sensually to demonstrate an inner state full of ecstasy. Visualize Kali as a young woman with long black hair and a sensual body. For this asana to be successful, you have to transform from submissive woman to a devourer. The great Kali pose is an icon for Tantra, since it represents the power of Eros and the feminine power of divinity.

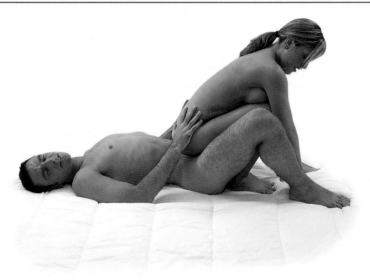

36 THE RABBIT

The man lies on his back and the woman squats with her back to him and moves with the lingam deep in her yoni.

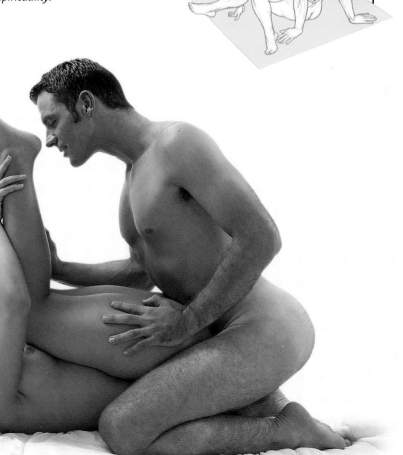

37 THE SACRED COUPLE

Both lovers visualize the journey of the kundalini from the sacrum to the head, and above, a shining golden circle where Shiva and Shakti meet. Correct breathing, visualization, *and meditation make the kundalini move upward, and the lovers will absorb divine qualities from the powerful visualization. This is the sacred alchemy of sexual energy into spirituality.*

137

38 THE BOW

Shakti, lying on her back, lifts both legs and holds her ankles. The man penetrates her yoni deeply.

39 UNITING THE FIRES
The woman lies flat and Shiva positions himself on top with his legs open, which allows him to feel feminine and active at the same time. He makes swaying and circular movement.

40 THE DRAGON
The man is on top of the woman and both their bodies feel totally united. This is a great position for relaxation.

41 FISH AGAINST FISH
Shiva bends his left leg and stretches out the right, which gives him balance. Shakti raises her right leg up and the left leg behind. This is a position that allows for deep penetration.

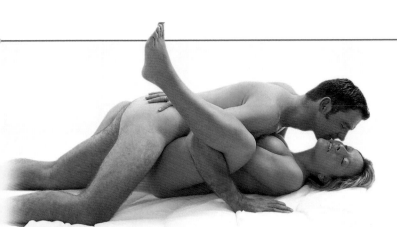

42 THREADING THE SILK
With the subtlety, dedication, and patience of artisan weavers at the loom, this position represents the soft fabric (Tantra) that the lovers make weaving the silk of love and meditative passion.

43 ENJOYING THE JEWEL
Shakti lies face down and Shiva positions himself on top. This allows two things: mutual relaxation and fusing of the chakras. Shiva's movements are slow and many Shaktis can reach orgasm when the man bites her neck, a highly erogenous zone.

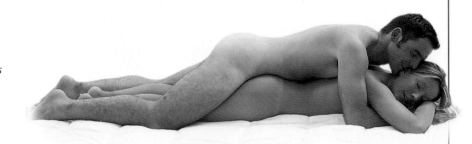

139

44 THE BRIDGE OF DESIRE
Shakti plants her feet while Shiva, with the force of his pelvis, lifts her a few centimeters off the ground. Her arms are outstretched above her head, suggesting openness. The man supports himself on his arms. The free movement comes from the goddess, who plays with her body, moving her hips.

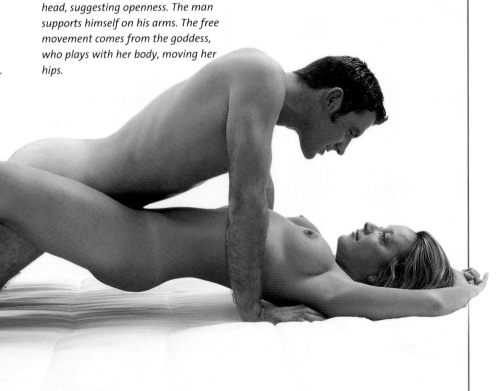

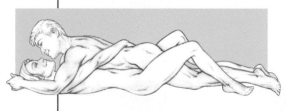

45 THE MISSIONARY

This is the only sexual position allowed for the "good" Christians, in which the man takes on an illusionary role of "superiority." Tantra doesn't recommend it too much because it favors ejaculation and literally squashes Shakti's body without allowing her to move. However, you can practice it slowly because some Shaktis like to feel covered by Shiva's body, and many reach orgasm from clitoral stimulation from Shiva's pubic hair.

46 THE WILD MARE

Seated on a chair, Shakti sits with her back to Shiva, who plays with her breasts (a highly erogenous zone) as if picking fruit from a tree. She also feels the support of his thighs. Her movements are powerful and free, moving her pelvis up and down.

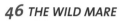

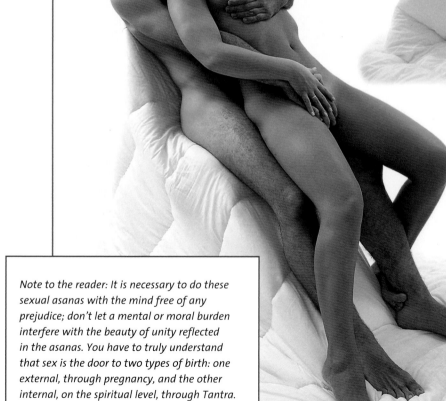

140

47 STIMULATING THE JEWELS

The man excites the goddess by gently touching her clitoris and nipples. This stimulation intensifies the body's bioelectricity. She leans against Shiva's body, who reclines in a chair, and assumes the passive role delighting in the magnetic touch of her lover's fingers. The meridians of energy begin and end in the fingertips, so contact with the jewels of the female body produce great pleasure. However, you shouldn't caress with them more than a few minutes, since they can become saturated and produce the opposite effect.

Note to the reader: It is necessary to do these sexual asanas with the mind free of any prejudice; don't let a mental or moral burden interfere with the beauty of unity reflected in the asanas. You have to truly understand that sex is the door to two types of birth: one external, through pregnancy, and the other internal, on the spiritual level, through Tantra.

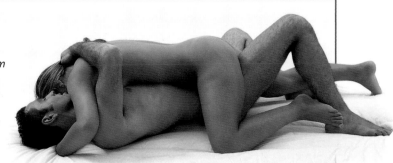

48 THE SACRED TRUTH

The goddess positions herself on top of Shiva, with her legs open, and fuses her chakras with his. This asana reveals the emotional and sexual superiority of the woman (her power on the sexual plane is seven times greater than man's). Tantra accepts this and gives the woman freedom to enjoy it and fulfill the sacred truth that "You must let the feminine dance above the masculine in liberty."

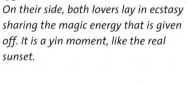

49 GOLDEN SUNSET

On their side, both lovers lay in ecstasy sharing the magic energy that is given off. It is a yin moment, like the real sunset.

50 THE UNIVERSAL FUSION

On top of Shiva, Shakti lays her hands on his. They breathe in unison and look at each other sweetly, fusing with the universal principles in total harmony and relaxation. The powerful bioenergetic currents nourish the couple on a physical, sexual, energetic, emotional, psychic, and spiritual level. Not in vain has Tantra revealed carnal love to be the road to the light in the soul.

141

51 THE PLEASURE OF TOUCHING THE JEWELS

Lying on the ground, the lovers give in to relaxation with a hand on their partner's organ. Breathe softly, visualize and feel the fine energy distributing from one body to the other. After maithuna, the lovers feel a strong magnetism that can allow them to experience astral journeys, or simply to enter the true temple of peace and divinity that lives inside the human heart.

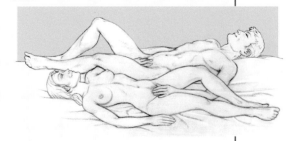

53 THE BOW

Like an arrow of energy shot into the whiteness of enlightenment, this bow formed by Shiva and Shakti is an invitation to fire arrows of serpentine fire with each breath. Shiva inhales and opens his chest when he goes back, and exhales softly when he goes forward.

52 THE SCISSORS

How beautiful is the possibility to share the "secret language" of Tantra. Shiva presses with his lingam when Shakti relaxes her yoni, and then the opposite. This language stokes the inner flame in the base of the first chakra. Moving as little as possible to maintain the temperature of maithuna, the lovers will press and relax their sexual organs for several minutes. The scissors also allows them to connect through the gaze, to discover that the lover is a mirror of light.

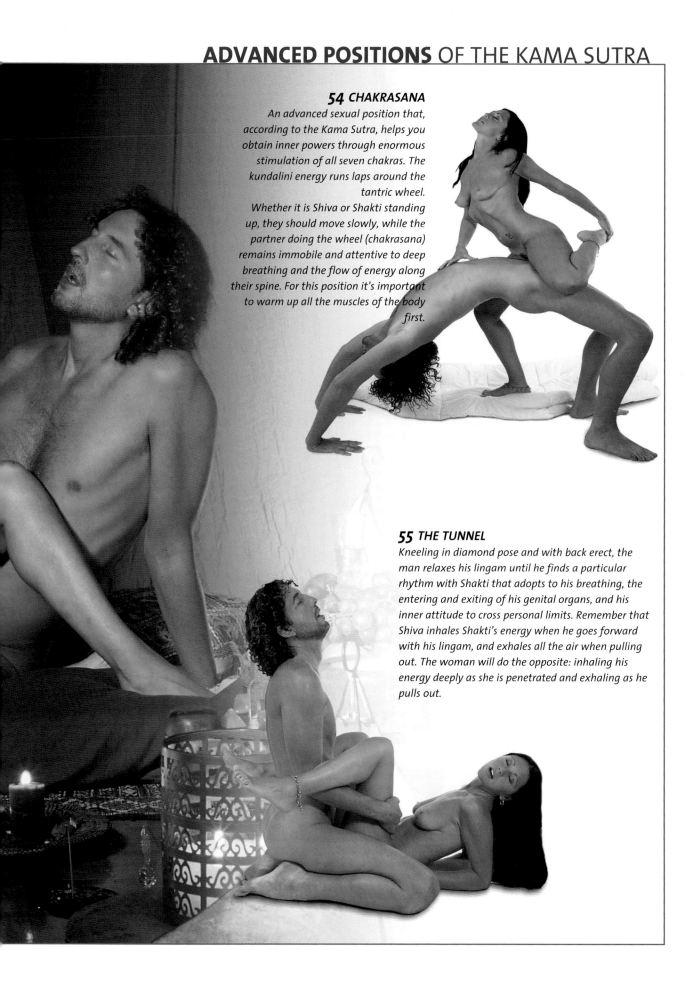

54 CHAKRASANA

An advanced sexual position that, according to the Kama Sutra, helps you obtain inner powers through enormous stimulation of all seven chakras. The kundalini energy runs laps around the tantric wheel.

Whether it is Shiva or Shakti standing up, they should move slowly, while the partner doing the wheel (chakrasana) remains immobile and attentive to deep breathing and the flow of energy along their spine. For this position it's important to warm up all the muscles of the body first.

55 THE TUNNEL

Kneeling in diamond pose and with back erect, the man relaxes his lingam until he finds a particular rhythm with Shakti that adopts to his breathing, the entering and exiting of his genital organs, and his inner attitude to cross personal limits. Remember that Shiva inhales Shakti's energy when he goes forward with his lingam, and exhales all the air when pulling out. The woman will do the opposite: inhaling his energy deeply as she is penetrated and exhaling as he pulls out.

56 THE TIGER ATTACKS FROM BEHIND

Tantric sexual practice contains waves of impulse, desire, ardor, passion, and wild force as well as peaks of relaxation, peace, stillness, bliss, and silence. This position incites the former, letting the animal instinct free, enjoying it, and overcoming it, traveling from base instinct to consciousness. The cadence is for the tiger, while the tigress gives in to the masculine power.

57 MOVEMENT OF THE ENERGETIC FIELD

For Tantra, the attraction between two people is due to their aura or energetic field. This position, which unites the chakras, is very important to connect, synchronize, and fuse the psyches, emotions, and bodies of the lovers. The man will be behind, penetrating with his lingam, and both partners remain completely still, breathing in unison and visualizing an enormous torrent of light, energy, desire, and consciousness that moves meditatively.

58 ROWING IN THE CURRENT

The goddess takes the boat of pleasure, with her back to Shiva, who lies face up. She can move her hips, sacrum, arms, and hair to the sound of passion and eros. Shiva can caress her back, but it is she who sets the rhythm, while he gives himself and fuses with the erotic joy of the feminine.

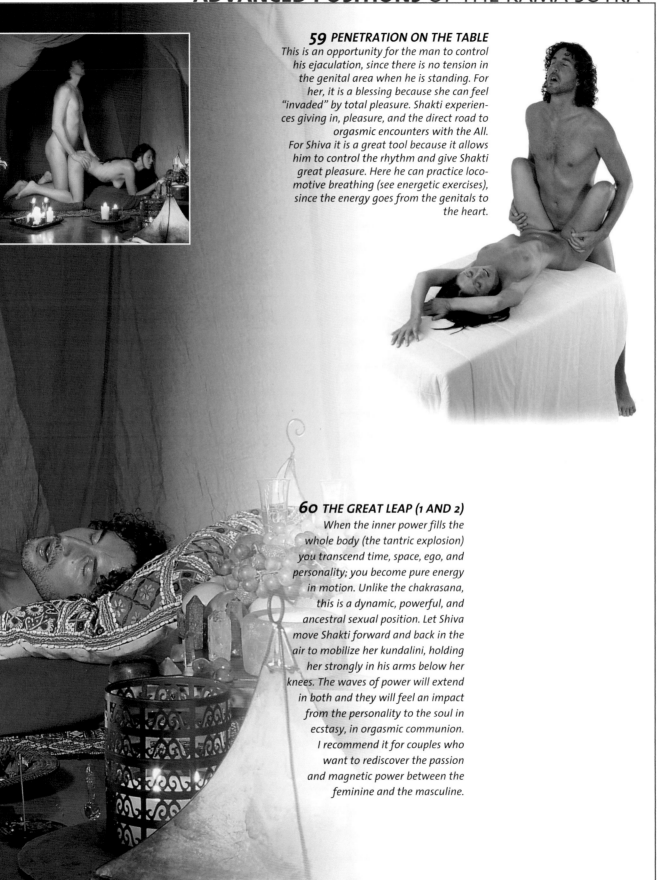

59 PENETRATION ON THE TABLE

This is an opportunity for the man to control his ejaculation, since there is no tension in the genital area when he is standing. For her, it is a blessing because she can feel "invaded" by total pleasure. Shakti experiences giving in, pleasure, and the direct road to orgasmic encounters with the All. For Shiva it is a great tool because it allows him to control the rhythm and give Shakti great pleasure. Here he can practice locomotive breathing (see energetic exercises), since the energy goes from the genitals to the heart.

60 THE GREAT LEAP (1 AND 2)

When the inner power fills the whole body (the tantric explosion) you transcend time, space, ego, and personality; you become pure energy in motion. Unlike the chakrasana, this is a dynamic, powerful, and ancestral sexual position. Let Shiva move Shakti forward and back in the air to mobilize her kundalini, holding her strongly in his arms below her knees. The waves of power will extend in both and they will feel an impact from the personality to the soul in ecstasy, in orgasmic communion. I recommend it for couples who want to rediscover the passion and magnetic power between the feminine and the masculine.

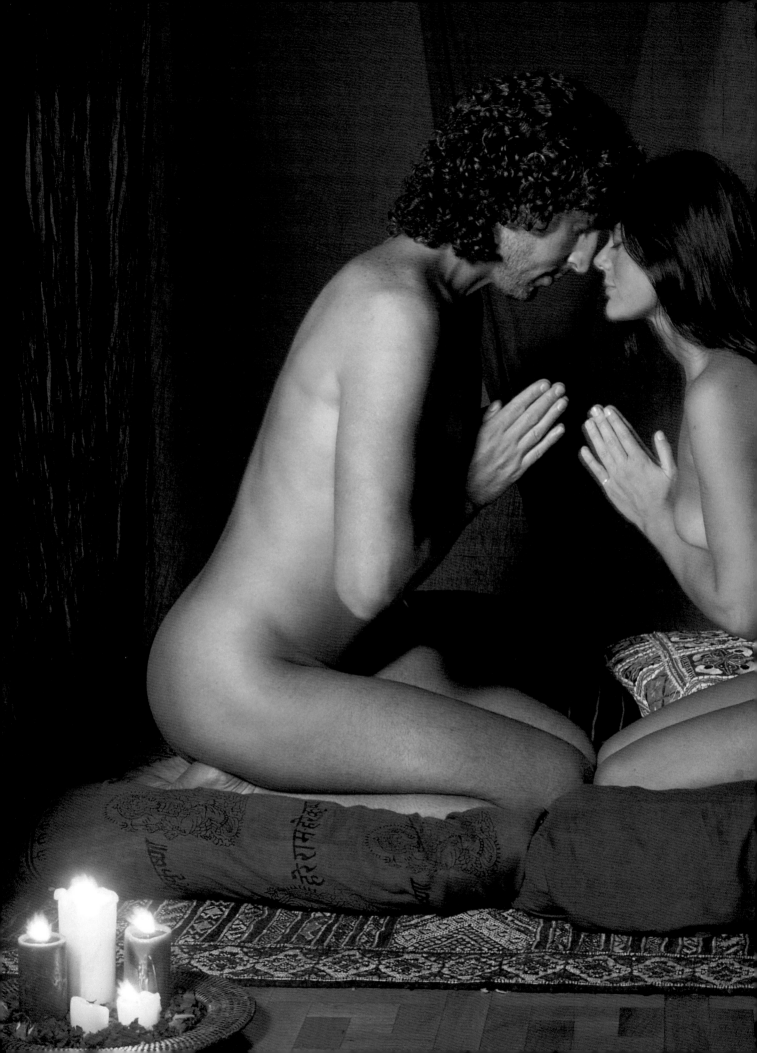

MAITHUNA:
THE MAGICAL SEXUAL ACT

*"Tantra has an ace of spades and that is maithuna,
the sexual ritual through which you fuse with your
partner in such a way that you lose all limits of body and soul.
It is an eternal moment when you experience the sacred spiritual unity."*
GUILLERMO FERRERA

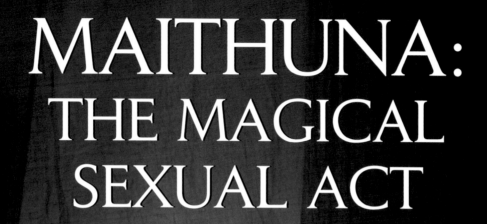

Steps to
ECSTASY

For Tantra, the orgasm is more than physical pleasure;
it is connection with the divine and access to the state of unity.
With the ritual of maithuna, sexual energy ascends through the
chakras and guides you to physical and spiritual joy.

For Tantra, the orgasm is more than physical pleasure; it is connection with the divine and access to the state of unity. With the ritual of maithuna, sexual energy ascends through the chakras and guides you to physical and spiritual joy.

Maithuna is the tantric consecration of woman and man to tune in, through sex, to the spiritual fountain within each of them. But it is also the opportunity to reach a state of unity where limits of duality disappear and the experience of ecstasy, the communion of bodies and souls, emerges.

Tantra develops the ritual of maithuna so that sexual energy leads to physical and spiritual pleasure. For Tantra, the orgasm is the connection to the divine, though the ascent of the kundalini in the sushumna and the seven chakras.

The brahamaranda, in the top of the head, opens to receive the kundalini that travels up from the sacrum. This is called the mystic matrimony: the cosmic wedding of Shiva and Shakti in the human body. Maithuna should be accompanied by conscious stimulation of the senses, so you should prepare a special environment that contains representations of the five senses.

THE ORDER OF THE RITUAL

The steps of maithuna are not rigid or automatic. Each couple will let their creativity flow freely, surprising their partner. I will describe a ritual that can be practiced by anyone who wants to start entering the magic world of Tantra.

It is important to think of it as a conscious game with which you will awaken vital, sexual, spiritual, and emotional energies in both partners with the goal of connecting in the inner spaces where the mind disappears and silence, peace, and ecstasy appear.

The way of Tantra through maithuna is a formidable invitation to eliminate boredom, awaken new sensations, prolong pleasure for hours, transform ejaculation into spiritual orgasm and creative energy, and bring the woman to liberation and joy.

But maithuna will also sweep clean a mind burdened with sexuality and fill it with spiritual sex, which is a pure experience of the body and spirit, of pleasure and meditation.

GOODBYE, MIND

The tantric experience of maithuna will be a journey you both enjoy from the body to the spirit, silencing the chatter of your mind along the way. This will suspend your intellectual and analytical activity, censorship, and conscience, which will guide the energy they awaken— consciousness of touching, of breathing, of penetrating and being penetrated, of feeling the energy in each chakra.

In maithuna you are at once the artwork and the artist. You both need to connect to your inner maestro, with the goddess and god you incarnate beyond time and identities.

The liberated energy will course through your sacred spaces, so you can reach a state of eternity, perception of the original androgyne, and the bridge to primordial unity.

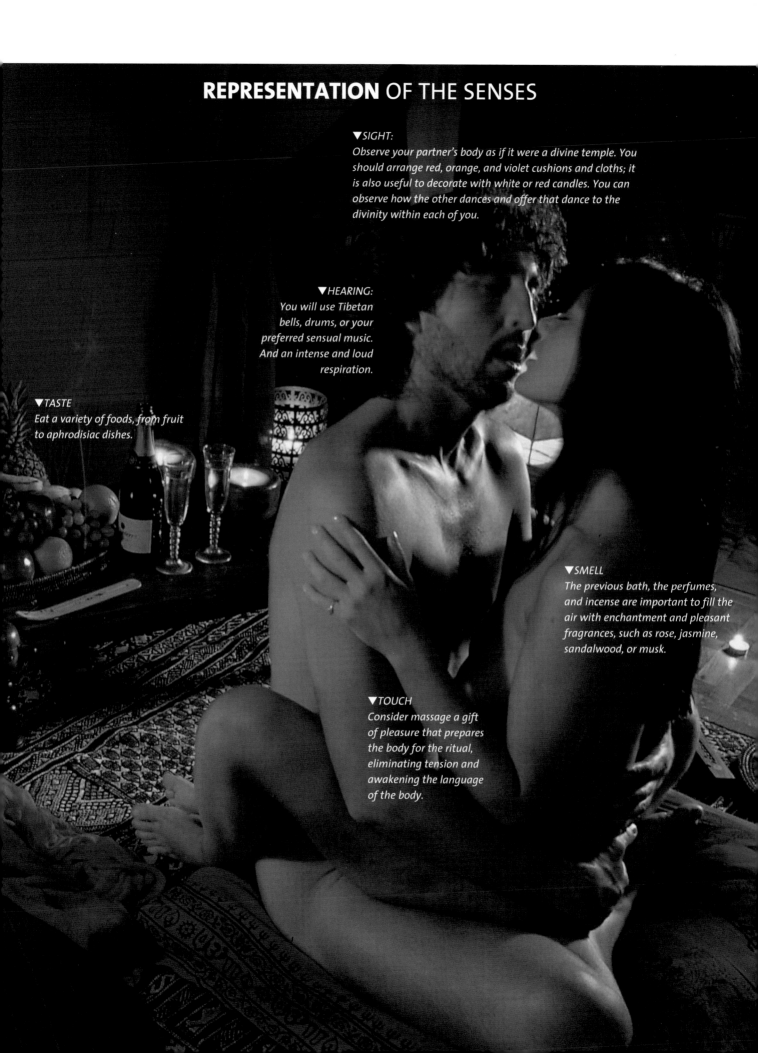

REPRESENTATION OF THE SENSES

▼SIGHT:
Observe your partner's body as if it were a divine temple. You should arrange red, orange, and violet cushions and cloths; it is also useful to decorate with white or red candles. You can observe how the other dances and offer that dance to the divinity within each of you.

▼HEARING:
You will use Tibetan bells, drums, or your preferred sensual music. And an intense and loud respiration.

▼TASTE
Eat a variety of foods, from fruit to aphrodisiac dishes.

▼SMELL
The previous bath, the perfumes, and incense are important to fill the air with enchantment and pleasant fragrances, such as rose, jasmine, sandalwood, or musk.

▼TOUCH
Consider massage a gift of pleasure that prepares the body for the ritual, eliminating tension and awakening the language of the body.

THE ORDER OF THE RITUAL

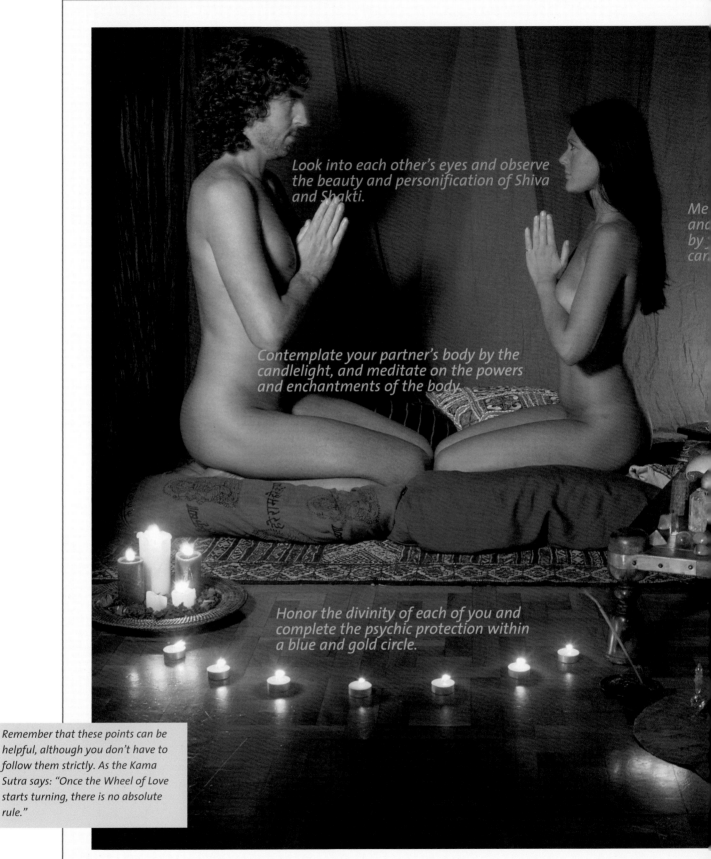

Look into each other's eyes and observe the beauty and personification of Shiva and Shakti.

Me
and
by
car.

Contemplate your partner's body by the candlelight, and meditate on the powers and enchantments of the body.

Honor the divinity of each of you and complete the psychic protection within a blue and gold circle.

Remember that these points can be helpful, although you don't have to follow them strictly. As the Kama Sutra says: "Once the Wheel of Love starts turning, there is no absolute rule."

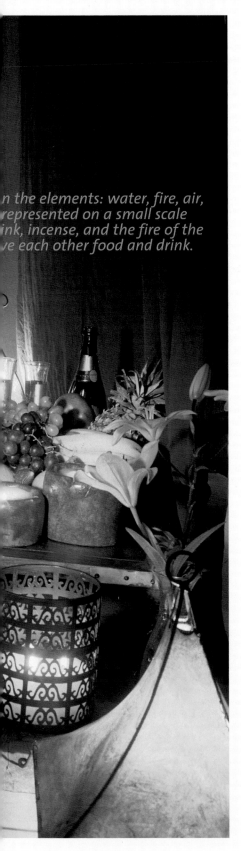

the elements: water, fire, air,
represented on a small scale
ink, incense, and the fire of the
e each other food and drink.

1. *Shower* or take an energetic or relaxing bath with salts.

2. *Remain conscious* of the magic act you will begin and start nyasa, the psychic protection.

3. *Decorate* the space with pillows and flowers, light candles and incense.

4. *Dance* for some minutes, give your dance to your lover, feeling that you are god and goddess.

5. *Look each other in the eyes*, observe the beauty and personification of Shiva and Shakti.

6. *Meditate on the elements:* water, fire, air, and earth, represented on a small scale by food, drink, incense, and the fire of the candles. Give each other food and drink.

7. *Contemplate your partner's body* by the candlelight, and meditate on the powers and enchantments of the body.

8. *Touch and kiss* each other's toes, buttocks, belly, chest, breasts, neck, cheeks, lips, eyes, forehead, and crown. Then do the same with the lingam and yoni.

9. *Massage* the body with aromatic oils.

10. *Breathe* deeply for several minutes, holding hands.

11. *Repeat the mantra OM* seven or nine times.

12. *Begin to make love* when you feel that the energy and passion are awakened.

13. *Hold back the climax* as many times as possible, just before reaching orgasm. This will make the experience stronger.

14. *Visualize* at all times how the shared energy rises along the spine.

15. At the moment of orgasm (or orgasms), *guide, with the inner eye,* the kundalini toward experiences of ecstasy, love, and spiritual enlightenment in the two highest chakras.

16. When you stop, it allows you to *absorb secretions* through the skin of the genitals, and then you will drink them, since they are highly energetic.

17. *Relax and meditate,* enjoying the silence, peace, and flow of energy through your body and psyche. This ritual can last from two to five hours, stopping to meditate and then beginning the sexual act again when the desire arises.

18. *Honor each other's divinity* and complete the psychic protection within a blue and gold circle.

151

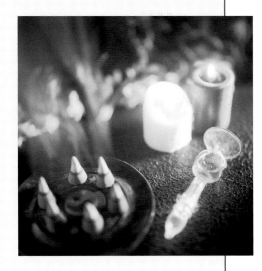

Seventh chakra
Absolute silence

Sixth chakra
OM

Fifth chakra
Ham

Fourth chakra
Yam

Third chakra
Ram

Second chakra
Vam

First chakra
Lam

SHIVA AND SHAKTI

The woman and man must take consciousness of the energy they incarnate. The woman will awaken all of her feminine energy (her Shakti, her inner goddess) and she will dance, first dressed and then naked, she will let her sensual and sexual impulse free, she will feel free, joyful, and ready to satisfy her desire. She will forget all repression and be her true self from the heart, connecting to the magic forces of nature and giving her body and soul to the man.

The man will feel the power of the masculine, of the dancer Shiva, and he will also dance. He will breathe vigorously to elevate his energy; he will touch his body and worship his lover's, whose energy he will feel through kisses and caresses. He will free himself from all control to feel fluid, open, and receptive, as if he traveled to nature's womb.

For Tantra there is no morality, nor room for prejudice, so it allows

> **The lovers should free themselves of prejudices and be conscious of the divinities they incarnate.**

you to share your energy with anyone, whether your life partner or someone you just met. This is because Tantra sees a Shakti in every woman, and a Shiva in every man, without names or personalities, and if there is attraction and the possibility of spiritual elevation then it won't deny the encounter. This is not a promotion of promiscuity or debauchery, just being conscious of desires and not repressing them. The encounter is, well, conscious of the factors that lead to two beings wanting to be united through sex.

In group tantric encounters, each woman leaves an object at the door, and each man chooses one at random; this is how he knows which woman he will do maithuna with. This explains that Tantra goes beyond the participants, centering on energy and sacred consciousness that you experience and overcoming the barriers of ego with its burden and prejudice.

DANCING

The lovers will let themselves be carried by the spell of special music and let the energy move through dance. They will do it naked, feeling in harmony with the dance of the universe and the planets, with the trees in the wind, and with all of Creation.

The dance is not just a simple dance; it is a meditative transport to awaken the bioenergy of the body and connect it to higher levels, where love, consciousness, and unity of opposites vibrate.

152

MANDALAS: MAKE YOUR OWN

A mandala is a concentric diagram, painting, or drawing that symbolizes order, center, and balance, and is used in tantric rituals to center psychic energies, whether cosmic or individual. You can make a mandala to concentrate on a certain point; this way concentration and respiration become a valuable formula to silence the mind. Although you don't need to do this together, it is positive because it allows your energies to unite.

BUILD YOUR MAGIC ENVIRONMENT
Prepare your meditation room and practice Tantra simply and specially: stimulate the senses, get comfortable, and try to make sure it is ventilated so prana from the Sun and air can enter. Prepare red, orange, violet, white, or garnet colored pillows and rugs, and unfold cushions and blankets. Light incense and perfume the air with essential oils; put out fresh flowers and decorate the walls with warm tones. Light white candles and put them around the room, or on a small table where you put the elements: earth, water, fire, and air symbolized by a small plant, a cup of water, the flame of a candle, and the smoke of incense. Prepare special music and keep aromatic oils on hand for massages. Enter barefoot as if it were a temple; don't allow arguments or bad energy. Fill the table with the gems for each chakra or some quartz crystals. You can make a small Feng Shui fountain where water flows between rocks. Have a basket of fruit and drinks. Let your creativity free to make it an oasis of pleasure and communication, where only enlightened souls enter.

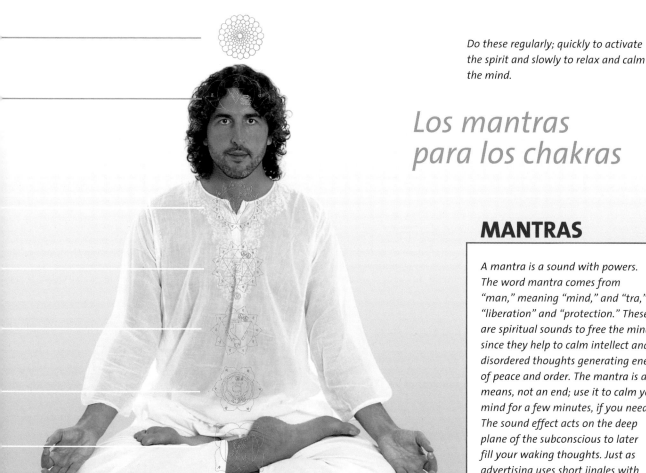

Los mantras para los chakras

MANTRAS

A mantra is a sound with powers. The word mantra comes from "man," meaning "mind," and "tra," "liberation" and "protection." These are spiritual sounds to free the mind, since they help to calm intellect and disordered thoughts generating energy of peace and order. The mantra is a means, not an end; use it to calm your mind for a few minutes, if you need to. The sound effect acts on the deep plane of the subconscious to later fill your waking thoughts. Just as advertising uses short jingles with catchy phrases that remain stuck in your head so you buy the product, a mantra acts so that the mind lets go of its contents.

The magic of the mantra soaks in best first thing in the morning, when its beneficial effects are freshest and most intense. However, you can also practice the mantras at any time, such as before going to sleep.

The sound OM is the mantra of the mantras, the sound of the universe. If you cover your ears and nose you can even hear it inside yourself, like a permanent echo. The "M" that mothers whisper to soothe their babies is natural wisdom, since it is a calming sound. Some mantras you can use are:

▼ *OM: the original primordial sound from which the universe was created; the sound of the sounds.*

▼ *OM MA NI PAD ME HUM: the jewel of the lotus is inside you.*

▼ *OM NAMA SHIVAYA: in the name of Shiva.*

▼ *SO HAM: "I am." Mentally repeat "So" with the inhalation and "Ham" with the exhalation.*

153

MEDITATION

After dancing freely and rubbing your bodies together, the lovers will sit face-to-face. They will control their breathing together, doing it slowly and deeply for at least ten minutes, then they will look each other in the eyes for a few more minutes to penetrate in their intimate essence.

Next, they will synchronize their breathing, letting it lead them deeper into the inner state. Breathing and feeling will be the love code that the tantric couple shares, but they won't only be united in breathing, body, and soul; their millions of sexual cells will also meet.

The breathing will allow the limits of the mind to dissolve, entering into a state of meditation where you capture the present, feel and perceive the All.

You can choose beforehand one of the meditations described in this book, and begin the sexual act itself when you are finished. Without any rush, the woman will play with the man's body, and he will play with hers. They will smell, touch, watch, listen to each other breathing, and delight in kisses and love bites. When they are ready, Shakti will invite Shiva to penetrate her, taking his lingam and inserting it in her yoni. Capturing the essence of unity at all times, they will breathe and begin to feel how the energies flow from one body to the other, forming the tantric circle. The sex act will be free and conscious, and every forty minutes they will do the "X" pose, consisting of holding hands while continuing with penetration; breathing and falling into the "Valley of Consciousness," a state of profound peace, relaxation, and unity.

Cuando la pareja t·ntrica
coge experiencia,
puede llegar al Èxtasis
llevando el deseo al
m·ximo o de forma
muy relajada.

THE ABRUPT PATH AND THE WAY OF THE VALLEY

Tantra uses two rhythms for the sexual act: the "Abrupt Path" and the "Way of the Valley." The first leads to maximum desire, since the man suspends his ejaculation and achieves orgasms without ejaculating and the woman is free to experience as many orgasms as she can, without limit but helping Shiva in the rhythms so that both go up the mountainside of desire and stop (breathing and halting all movement) until the energy leaves the lingam and disperses. The blood will leave the lingam and it will shrink a little, then start over again. The Abrupt Path is like climbing a mountain without ever reaching the peak.

The Way of the Valley is the road where you never reach a crescendo of desire, but rather do the sex act very slowly. With almost imperceptible movements, the lovers enjoy the sensations in total relaxation.

Once the tantric couple gains experience, they can visit both paths since they are totally compatible, just that the first reaches orgasm through excitement and the second, through relaxation.

WHAT HAPPENS WITH ENERGY IN THE BODY?

When the kundalini begins to mobilize along the energetic channels, the link between Shiva and Shakti is extremely powerful.

For Traditional Chinese Medicine (such as acupuncture, digipuncture, and shiatsu) there are two energetic

FIVE WAYS TO KISS

The kiss is contact to awaken energy. When two mouths and tongues touch, it automatically awakens sexual energy. The tongue is linked to the sexual center. Tantra is romantic and scientific at the same time, since it unites love and intelligence, and so it proposes five ways to kiss in order to awaken sexual energy.

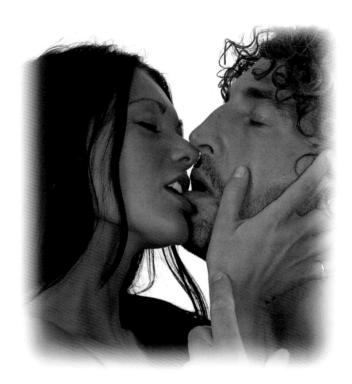

1. Love bites. Softly bite your lover's lips, delicately but passionately, to awaken the animal instinct. You have to play with love bites as if you were two tigers loving each other before copulating.

channels, called the governing vessel (GV) and the conception vessel (CV). These channels go from the sexual area to the top of the head, descending along the center of the forehead to the upper lip, and then from the lower lip back to the sexual area passing over the chest and navel. This course is important not only for Tantra but for all the spiritual and energetic ways of the East.

Awakened energy can be channeled along these paths so that both energetic principles, positive and negative, unite to give birth to light.

Tantra will make you and your partner a unit of energy, love, and communication. It is the intelligent and pragmatic way that leads a human being

to understand his or her self and all those around him or her, since whoever transforms their sexual energy becomes a powerful, radiant, and creative being.

The energy will travel along the CV and GV with breathing, visualization, and inner power. Practice this technique for five to ten minutes.

WHEN TO STOP?

For Tantra, time does not exist in maithuna, which can be enjoyed from two to five hours, with intervals of relaxation, meditation, visualization, and special breathing. What's more, every time you practice it the sensations will be different.

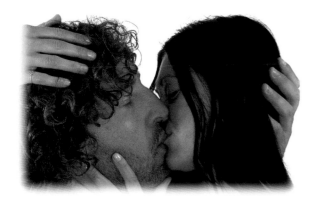

2. Lip kiss. *Contact from lip to lip.*

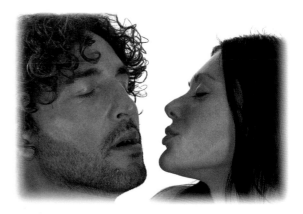

3. Blowing. *Blow gently to tickle the mouth and neck.*

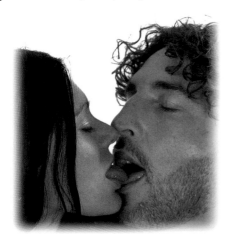

4. Tongue kiss. *The tongues touch each other and the other's lips. With his kiss, energy awakens in the genitals immediately.*

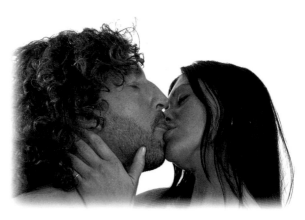

5. Suction kiss. *With your lips, alternate taking the upper or lower lip of your partner and suck gently.*

When you feel that energy has bathed you in light, vitality, consciousness, and creativity, you can finish the maithuna by bringing your hands to your chest and saluting the divinity of your lover, giving thanks for so much pleasure. You can stop every forty minutes and practice the "X" pose in order to consecrate the maithuna by using sexual magic, concentrating all your awakened energy on a special project, such as increasing the level of love, sending light to the planet, deepening the energetic and spiritual state, going on astral journeys, or whatever you need as a couple.

WHEN DOES THE MAN EJACULATE?

Don't feel guilty if at first you can't control ejaculation. Instinct and habit have formed a downward path for energy. Don't worry, enjoy it. The art of not ejaculating takes time, and when you learn the trick you will feel how your body assimilates the accumulated energy. Don't let yourself fill with tension, remember to use the energy creatively.

ASVINI MUDRA

To awaken the kundalini and make it rise in hot waves from the first chakra, you should practice asvini mudra occasionally. It consists of practicing good breathing technique while you contract and relax the anal sphincter (twenty to forty times) to generate heat in that area and incite the energy to follow the path set by your consciousness. This way, the PC muscle is strengthened, allowing the man to transform his ejaculation into ojas shakti, and the woman to strengthen her orgasms.

SPECIAL BREATHS

You don't have to reach the point of imminent ejaculation to practice special breaths; you can do these at any time to expand both energy and level of consciousness. I recommend you practice the breaths during daily sadhana in order to know which to use during maithuna. Depending on the circumstances, you may use different techniques.

1. Locomotive breaths
Inhale and exhale rapidly through the mouth for two or three minutes; as if you were an animal panting. This allows the energy to leave the genital area and the sound will excite the lovers. Do it now and then to control energy.

2. Bellow breaths
Inhale and exhale rapidly through the nose; like a bellow that stokes the fire, your nose will send more air and prana to the serpentine fire of the kundalini. Do this occasionally for two or three minutes.

3. Heart breaths
Inhale and exhale through the mouth very slowly, but deep and loud, letting out a big "Aaaahhhh." Concentrate the energies on your heart to bring the kundalini to the heart chakra and awaken the experience of eternal love. This should last about ten minutes, but stop if you feel dizzy.

This is a powerful breathing technique that will make the physical body feel more subtle and ethereal, and your energetic field like waves of electric energy in motion.

4. Chakra breaths
At the same rhythm, do seven breaths for each chakra, inhaling through the nose and exhaling through the mouth. You can do this back-to-back to feel the heat and energy emanating from the chakras.

5. Complete breaths to elevate the kundalini
Both of you synchronize with the same cadence of breathing, visualizing the kundalini like a tube of orange light that circulates from the first to the seventh chakra. This way the energetic orbits become very powerful and magnetized.

You can ejaculate once every eight or ten sexual acts, or in winter, once every fifteen times. Conserve your semen (bindu) as much as you can, but don't think of it as a race or a challenge. With daily practice of sadhana before maithuna, you will be able to prevent ejaculation naturally. But if ejaculation does happen, breathe a few times contracting the anal sphincter in asvini mudra, visualize your energy (some of it stays in the body and you won't lose as much vitality), and dedicate it to the sensual spirit of the cosmic Shakti. You can also do it on the nights of a full moon to enjoy the spirit of Kali and transmute energy, filling yourself with tremendous power.

THE GODS LOVE EACH OTHER CONSCIOUSLY . . . AND CONSCIOUS LOVERS BECOME GODS!

Tantra is a manual of wisdom; a way without footprints that transforms your life into a blessing. Everything, both bad and good, makes sense.

The possibility that Tantra offers to mortal men and women is that of awakening, feeling, experiencing, and enjoying the divine essence that they have inside. The earthly culmination of the tantric road, enlightenment, comes from any of the tantric practices (pranayamas, meditations, and sexual maithuna).

You will not be the same person after practice, since you will be more enlightened. Just as there is light in a light bulb the same as in the Sun, your unique being has light the same as Jesus, Buddha, Krishna, Osho, or Zaratustra, although to a different degree.

You have the key to elevate your level of light day by day: you are special! With Tantra you will reach the metaphysical experience of feeling your transpersonal space, where God lives making your heart beat and filling your consciousness.

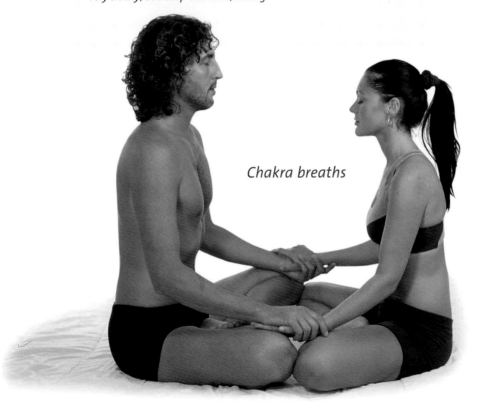

Chakra breaths

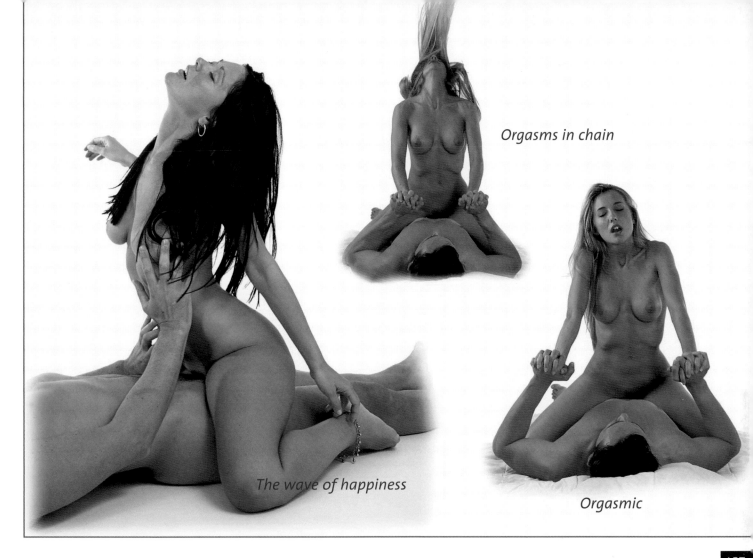

Orgasms in chain

The wave of happiness

Orgasmic

USE OF SEXUAL MAGIC

Sexual energy is magical, and magic can be used in a white, black, or red way. This book encourages you to center on Light, the powerful white magic, knowing that everything we give to the universe comes back multiplied. (And who wants darkness in return?)

Tantra is a way of light that teaches us that sexual magic can be useful to create higher bodies and spiritual states. The physical, energetic, emotional, and mental bodies are created by nature; but the spiritual, cosmic, and nirvanic bodies are found in a latent state in all of us, so it is the responsibility of the individual to create them for his or her self. The compensation is enormous; nothing more and nothing less than consciousness of eternity, and the return to the cosmic home.

FIVE LEVELS OF ORGASM

All women and men are born with the capacity to orgasm. Tantra teaches that the orgasm is a state of physical and spiritual communion; the loss of the mind, and the return to the innocence, joy, and pleasure from which we were created. It is a natural state of life, since life flows in an orgasmic nature. The raw material of the universe is ecstasy and the sexual act is contact with this vibration. The man should seek to bring his partner to orgasm quickly and repeatedly. Tantra lists five levels of orgasmic pleasure:

1. Preorgasmic
When the energy prepares to be distributed. (You can't always reach the second level from here.)

2. Occasional
When you can achieve orgasm but not every time, whether it's because of physical or emotional tension, having a bad day, receiving bad news, etc.

3. Orgasmic
The state in which most men and women feel satisfied.

4. Orgasms in chain
Couples reach this level when they let themselves be carried away by desire, into the skies of freedom.

5. The wave of happiness
Potent and quality orgasms extended in time. This is the home of the tantrics, both men and women.

THE SECRET LANGUAGE

> *Shiva and Shakti have a communication code during maithuna called "the secret language." It is the alternating pressure and relaxation of the lingam and yoni. The woman presses with her yoni when the man relaxes his lingam; then the man presses his lingam and the woman relaxes her yoni. This awakens the kundalini that both will later drive through visualization.*
>
> *The best positions for the secret language are the "X" laying down and the Shiva-Shakti seated. Practice the secret language for a few minutes.*

Sexual energy can be the motor to create these bodies or states of expanded consciousness, as well as to develop the powers of telepathy, clairvoyance, spiritual awakening, and intuitive perception. But all magic needs a mage and Tantra will make you someone who knows that the way of magic is the way of life. The magic power awakens in tantric practice and initiates you in its ways.

The accumulation of climax without reaching orgasm produces magical energy. Shakti can reach orgasm, the tantric wave of happiness, but the man should not ejaculate, but rather transform it into orgasm. In the moment that she climaxes, he should close his eyes and ride the wave with her: close the muscles of the anal sphincter, hold his breath and look upward to center his consciousness on the seventh chakra. He can also bring his tongue to his palate or press with two fingers on the point between the anus and the lingam to not ejaculate.

This allows both to exchange subtle energy and the electricity produced will make both bodies vibrate in magic currents, so that the physical consciousness disappears and spiritual consciousness emerges. The climax of sex becomes divine ecstasy, but the wave doesn't end there: after a rest, Shakti will rise again, because the whirlwind of energy is very strong. The orgasms of both the woman and man will reach ever-higher peaks, so the man needs great control to not end desire or ejaculate.

The tantric yogi lets himself be carried by the energy of his partner, and she by his power, as both rise to the peaks of pleasure and consciousness.

When the energy rises, it moves through the chakras, and sexual magic makes the kundalini run through the chakras and purifies emotions. You must pay close attention and be conscious in every moment.

Sexual magic can be used to make a wish come true, so both partners should visualize what they most desire in the moment of orgasm. For this magic to work, it's important to know the secrets of breathing, since the magic fire is carried upward by visualization and conscious breathing.

The magic energy is employed by breathing for each of the chakras while you visualize its color and mantra. Then, the energy is stored in the muladhara chakra or the Third Eye, and will provide inspiration to be used in the creation of the higher bodies, or simply whenever needed.

The lingam will be a magical source of spirituality and pleasure, and the yoni a recipient of magic secrets. These practices are rejuvenating, and the tantric couple will open doors to sexual secrets and the chakras.

MAGIC WITH THE FULL MOON

The Moon is an ancestral magical object. It represents fertility, mystery, the energies of the night, poetic inspiration, and the awakening of the mystical.

To silence the mind, you can spend a few minutes repeating the mantra OM, the mantra of the Moon (LAM), or the following prayer:

*"Queen of the Night,
you have been through time
and space,
show me the secrets of life
so I can feel unity with all
the universe.*

*Queen of inspiration,
come to me with your energy of love,
so my soul transcends all limits
and I know the sublime."*

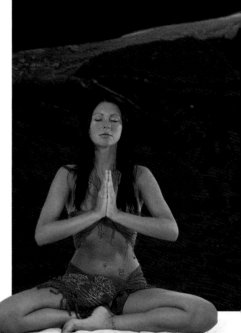

With hands united at your chest, take a deep inhalation.

The Sun represents the diurnal polarity, so the Moon, which reflects the light of the Sun, is the nocturnal polarity.

In silence, the couple will connect to the lunar energies. They will sit or lie down in a meditation pose, letting the moonlight touch their naked bodies, and they will breathe for several minutes so that the human consciousness connects to the magic consciousness.

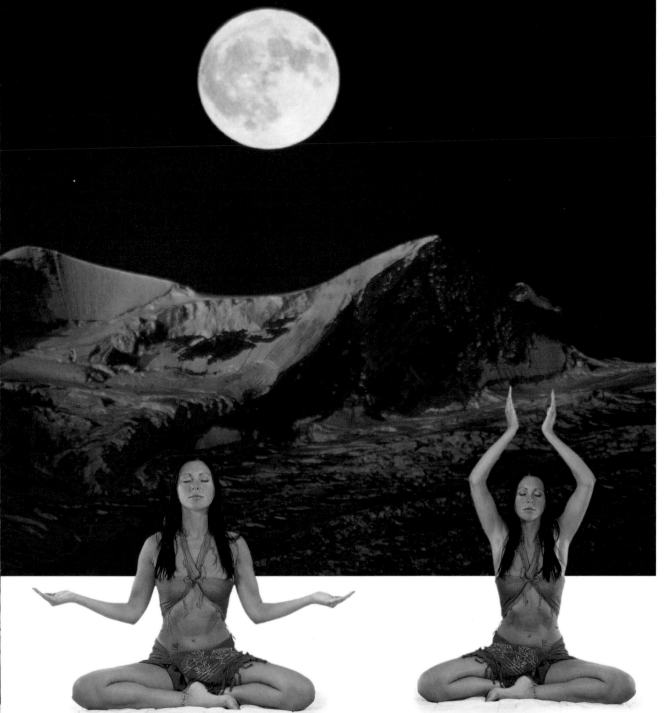

Lift your arms above your head to form a circle.

Bring your palms together at the top and lower them once more to your chest, to begin again.

Then, seated, they will do the exercise diagramed above.

This breathing is done with consciousness focused on taking energy from the Moon—whether you are looking at it through a window, in the open air in a forest, or near the sea (something very beautiful and powerful.)

Do this focusing the entrance of energy on two chakras: from the top of the head, to the heart. All magic comes from the heart.

The couple needs a purpose, whether it is accumulating energy, creating an energetic body like a cosmic egg, sending energy long distance, deepening the state of consciousness, going on astral journeys (best while lying down in shavasana), or whatever other thing the couple needs.

Magic work is a movement of energy, and this is what tunes in, when it rises, to the magic dimension of life. This dimension is reality, the Absolute that creates and recreates in every moment.

Life dances magically, everything that happens has a magic stamp and, sooner or later, we will all find ourselves dancing to the same eternal song as the divine.

MAGIC WITH THE SUN

Lying in shavasana on the ground, with head pointing toward the Sun, take deep breaths in, imagining that the solar energy enters your head and goes down to your feet.

Then, in the exhalation, imagine that the energy of the earth enters your feet and goes up to your head. The going down of the Sun and the rising of the earth will unite the earthly and the divine within you.

After a few minutes, bring all the energy to the heart, where you will visualize a powerful and luminous circle for at least half an hour. Then, sit and breathe to charge the solar chakra.

The purpose is the same as before. You can also repeat the mantra RAM (the mantra of the Sun) or OM, or fill your consciousness with the following prayer:

"Light of beginnings, light of days,
which the Egyptians, Indians, and Mayans
adored,
to which we all owe devotion,
fill my heart with power and love."

"King Star, whose kingdom of light is before us,
I give you thanks for your energy and for
guiding the way of light.
May your fire awaken in my spirit and fill it with
dance.
May your fire burn away the impure so my soul
will shine."

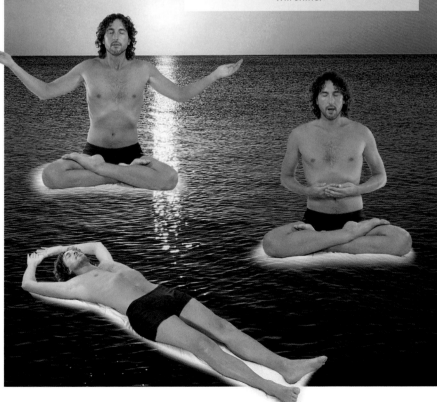

MAGIC WITH FIRE

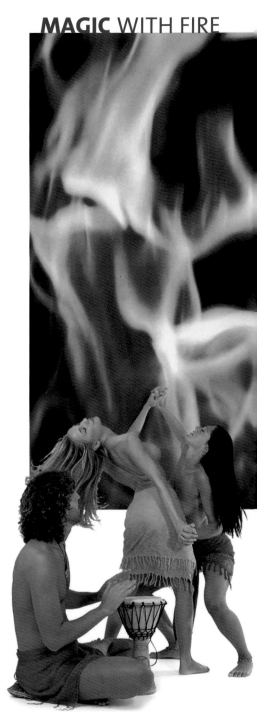

First phase

1. Dance with your naked body around the flames. If you do it with your partner or a group of people, the effect is increased.

2. Breathe energetically, visualizing and feeling that the qualities of the fire awaken the inner fire and lift it.

3. Play drum music.

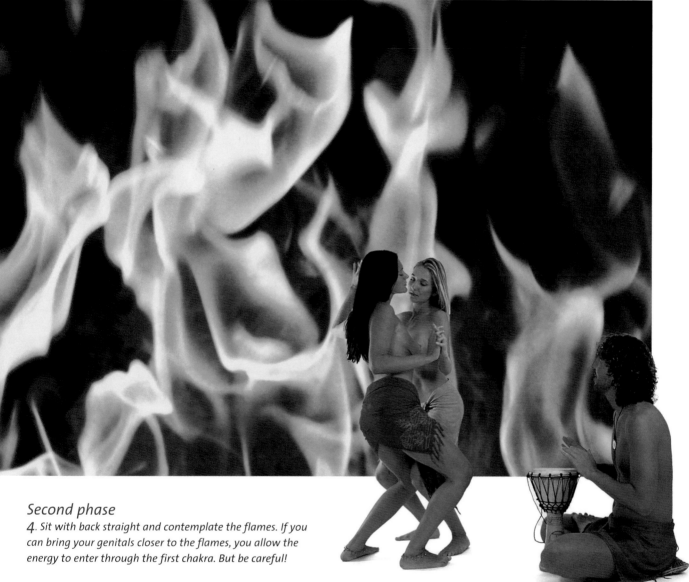

Second phase

4. Sit with back straight and contemplate the flames. If you can bring your genitals closer to the flames, you allow the energy to enter through the first chakra. But be careful!

5. Close your eyes and listen to it crackle, while you visualize how the fire burns within you. Breathe energetically and deeply for at least fifteen minutes, so that the energy mobilizes. Inhale through the nose and exhale through the mouth.

6. You can invoke your personal god and visualize a wish for your soul's evolution, feeling the fire in your heart. Resume breathing softly and calmly.

Third phase

7. Lie back in silence to listen to the crackle of the flames and exterior silence. At this point, your consciousness will be totally fused and connected to the fire.
Don't put the fire out with earth or water; wait until it burns out completely.

The fire has been used as a magic tool to connect with the invisible and mystic side of nature. Our ancestors worshiped fire in ceremonies and rituals, dancing, meditating, leaping, and entering into a trance so that the luminous spirits granted wisdom.

Within the body, the fire element represents action, spiritual energy, enthusiasm, faith, and sexual energy. This inner fire grows from the air generated by yogic breathing to burn off impurities and manifest the soul clearly. The inner fire is centered in the solar chakra, in the mouth of the stomach. If the fire of the kundalini (in the first chakra) awakens, it will send energy to all the chakras, to the eyes, the brain, the organs, and the cells, and will illuminate the divine characteristics of each person.

EXERCISES IN SACRED SEXUALITY

1. Penetration in stages

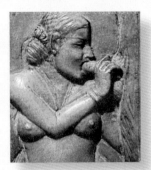

After sucking on the glans, Shakti takes in the lingam to a third of its length, then two-thirds, and then all of it.

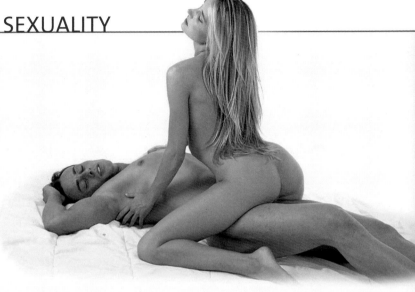

2. *Movements you should avoid are strong movements from the waist and any brusque movements; especially deep thrusts of the lingam. It is beneficial to* **maintain pubis to pubis contact** *to stimulate the clitoris.*

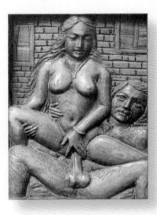

First, Shakti positions herself on top of Shiva, opens the lips of her vulva and presses it against the shaft of the lingam, while Shiva relaxes (especially in the abdomen and buttocks) and breathes deeply. Shakti, with discrete swaying movements, slides her vulva (clitoris included) along the lingam, sometimes to the point of orgasm.

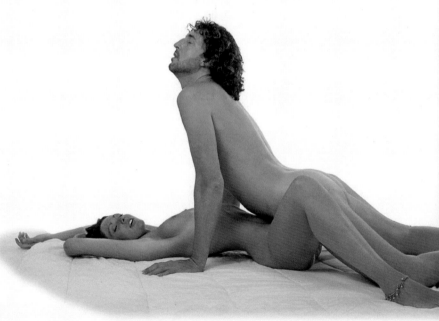

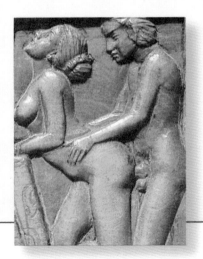

Immobile and with the senses awake, the lovers remain attentive to what happens between them. They open themselves to intimate, amorous fusion, without caresses or any other movement that could increase the sexual tension. There is no thrusting, just the "secret language" (pressing of the yoni and the lingam).

162

3. Shiva should practice mula bandha, or the contracting of the muscles of the anus, so when he approaches the limit he can relax them; this will decrease the erection and the tension, and the experience continues. Then he must contract them again, to relax them later.

If Shiva observes his own reflexive behavior when approaching ejaculation, he will notice, in addition to a quickening of rhythm and breathing, a strong tension in the muscles of the buttocks, abdomen, lower back, and lingam, and if he lets go (as is habitual), it will let loose the ejaculatory reflex, in which all these muscles participate. In order to delay or impede ejaculation, he must control his breathing and all these muscles. As a result, his movements will be more flexible and harmonious, and his rhythm will be more pleasant for Shakti.

PRINCIPLES
OF MAITHUNA

1. Don't try to achieve anything
2. Enjoy the pleasure without clinging to it
3. Be conscious of the energy at all times
4. Forget ego and feel the sacred principles in each of you
5. Unite the inner Shiva and Shakti
6. Let your breathing be the bridge to cross from the mundane to the sacred
7. Allow the mind to stop working and remain in silence

EXERCISES IN SACRED SEXUALITY

4. To effect ejaculation, control exhalation.

First of all, you must remain very calm during the entire union (especially when approaching the limit) and concentrate on the experience, remaining conscious of your breathing at all times. In the current union, the rhythm of breathing and coital motions synchronize spontaneously so that the push produces exhalation and the pulling out, inhalation. While sailing on calm waters, far from the point of limit, he can keep this sequence. Shiva has two options: inverting this rhythm when close to the limit (push: inhalation, pulling out: exhalation) or he can adopt a slow, deep, even breathing during the whole contact.

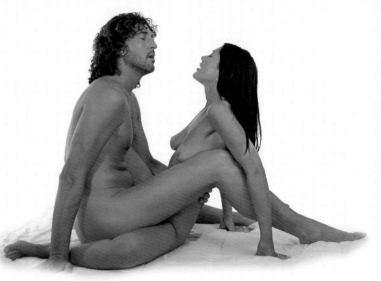

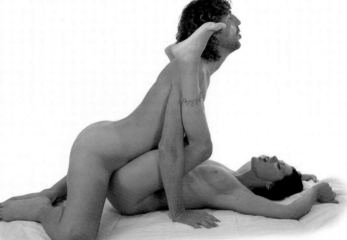

5. When approaching the point of limit, he can *do the jiva bandha*: fold the tongue against the palate and push it back as far as possible.

6. If the instinct to ejaculate appears, *do two minutes of locomotive breaths*, through the mouth and very dynamically, until the genital tension is reduced and the energy is distributed all through the body.

7. If the man feels that ejaculation is imminent, he should press his left index and middle finger on *the acupuncture point located a few centimeters above the right nipple*, while exhaling all the air through the nose. This will stop the emission of semen and raise the energy to his head, providing inner power. Another technique is to *press the point situated between the anus and the genitals*, so that the ejaculation goes back and nourishes the body. This is an internal ejaculation and can channel energy to the spine and the chakras.

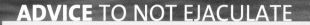

ADVICE TO NOT EJACULATE

1. Don't get too excited—go toward climax and stop
2. Do three gentle penetrations for every deep penetration
3. Establish a slow rhythm, especially at the beginning
4. Breathe consciously at all times
5. Control the movements of the mind
6. Bring your tongue to your palate
7. Use any of the techniques described before climax to avoid the loss of energy
8. Use asvini mudra and mula bandha; control of the anal sphincter
9. Stop every forty minutes and breathe to exchange bodily fluids

165

CONCLUSION

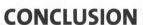

Tantra is the awakening of consciousness and heart; a feeling so immense that it frees us and connects us to life itself.

Sometimes when we are alone before the sea or a mountain, making love, or meditating, we have the sensation of spiritual connection. Other times, a person, a song, a book, a creative activity, or something special can be the bridge to the center of your being.

The Mahanirvana Tantra says: "Fish, meat, grains, roots, fruits, and any other thing offered ritually to the higher kingdoms, along with wine, are called 'ingredients of worship.' Let each one raise a glass and meditate on the kundalini. She is the pure energy that travels from the sexual center to the tip of the tongue. When the kundalini is excited, rises, and reaches the center of the head, bliss emerges from the encounter between her and the Moon of the consciousness."

This inner center is the essence from which Tantra wants you to live. In this world, we learn to feel deeply, so it is important from day to day to connect to this spring of energy and express it creatively. When you open your heart, the mystic and joy of living emerge passionately, and you experience happiness. But Tantra is not free, you must pay a price: daily energetic practice and use of consciousness. The result will be the rediscovery of magic, wonder, an inner space full of enthusiasm, and cherishment of the present. When you feel this wave of bliss, your life becomes a work of art, lived fully. As Osho said: "With the happiness of Zorba and the deepness of Buddha."

I am sure this book will help you understand the particular and holistic focus on the human being that Tantra has. I'm also sure that the perfume of your practice will be the joy of living life as an adventure, the acceptance and discovery of who you are.

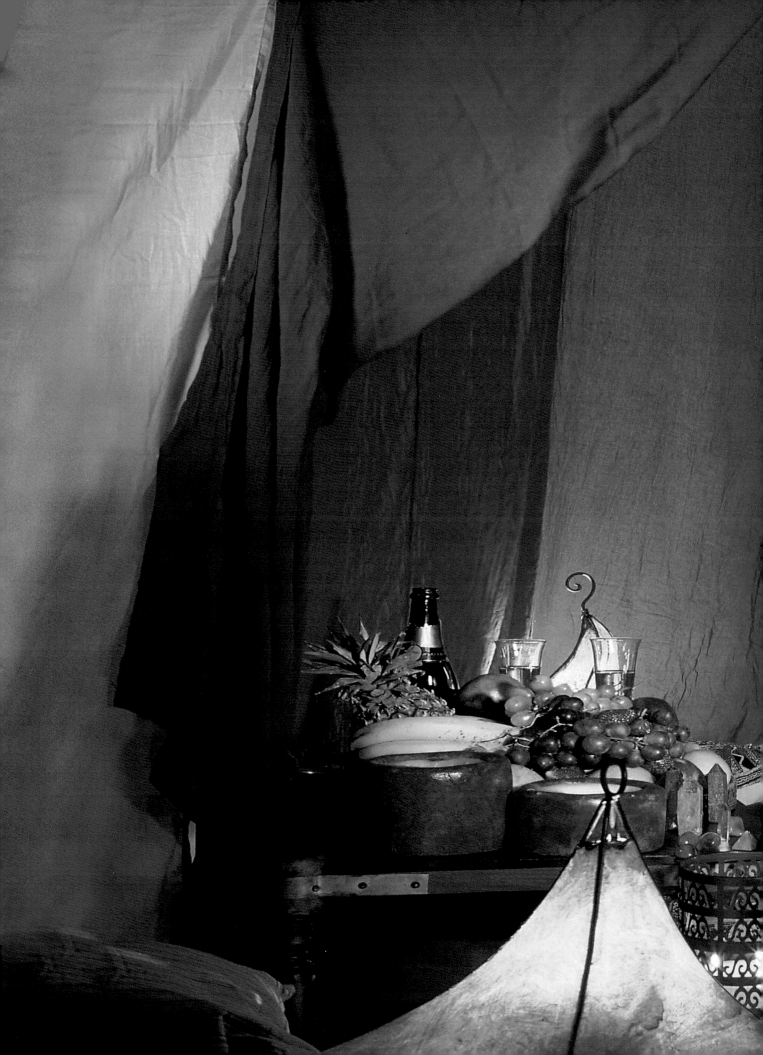

TANTRIC
RITUALS

*"Life is magical;
children are connected to the Magic of Life.
To be a Mage, you must be innocent like a child."*

Ritual of
SHIVA AND SHAKTI

The sacred encounter of man and woman transcends physical union to reach the divine.

The "lovers" ("two who love," whether married or not) choose a special night when they both know they won't be interrupted, and begin the ritual.

First of all, they should take a shower or bath with salts, but not for more than twenty minutes. Then, they dress in light clothing; preferably white or gold for the man (representing day and the Sun) and black for the woman (like the darkness of the night). They go to the room prepared for the act. Preferably the rituals should be done on a floor covered with carpets, pillows, and cushions, and welcoming decorations—flowers, candles and incense, small gifts, baskets of fruits and nuts, spirits or juices.

The couple will begin the ceremony thusly:

1 Closing their eyes, they visualize a white circle or fire around them. This circle can be made mentally, or physically with candles, flower petals, a rope, or chalk.

2 Standing, with consciousness awakened, the woman slowly recites:

"I am Shakti, the goddess / I am feminine power, movement, fertility / I am like the water between the rocks. I am Shakti, the holy, the giver of life / I am the girl, the woman, the mother, the wise, the magic, and the old / I am the beginning of life.

I receive you, oh Shiva, man, god / my husband, my hero. / More than your name is your essence that I worship with devotion."

3 Greeting with palms together at the chest, she will let her partner recite the following:

"I am Shiva, the god, / I am the dance of life / I am the masculine power, I am the light and spiritual impulse, / I am like the fire that dances with flames toward the sky. I am Shiva, the passion of existence / I am the boy, the man, the father, the wise, the magic, the patriarch / I am the spark that lights destinies.

I receive you, oh Shakti, woman, goddess / my companion, my dancer. / More than

your name is your essence that I worship with devotion."

4 Greeting with pranava mudra, hands on the chest, the lovers look into each others eyes a few moments, put on drum music, and repeat: "I give you my dance." They begin to move freely, breathing deeply and slowly, allowing the dance to mobilize the energy of the bodies.

5 As their body heat rises, they let their clothing fall gently within the circle, offering nakedness of the body and soul. They dance naked without touching for ten or fifteen minutes.

6 They sit face-to-face, backs straight and legs crossed in ardha siddhasana or half lotus, and look each other in the eyes in the flickering candlelight, with devotion and love.

7 Taking each other's hands, they begin Shiva–Shakti pranayama: they bring their noses close without touching and when one inhales, the other exhales.

OBJECTIVE

Unifying of consciousness. Feeling of unity. Samadhi. Crossing the borders of ego, time, and space. Doing Magic to fulfill a wish. Connection with the eternity of the present moment.

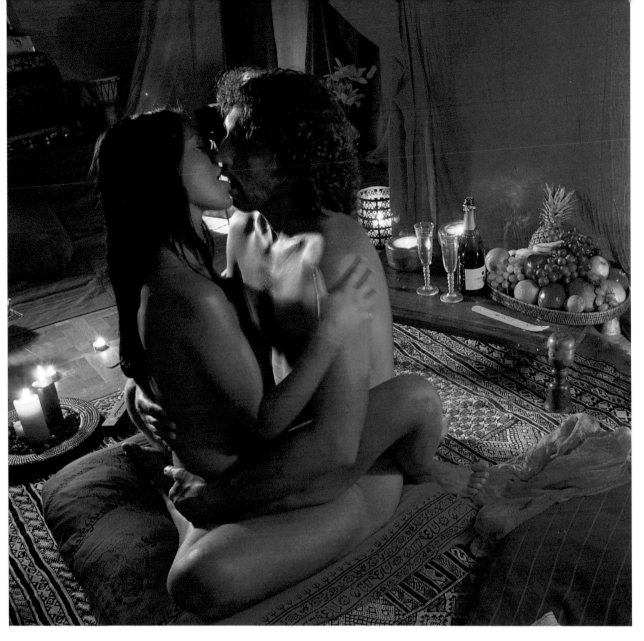

The rituals require a comfortable and pleasant setting: cushions, candles, and incense are some of the fundamental ingredients for a welcoming feel.

They breathe the air their lover exhales for at least fifteen minutes, and then recite the mantra OM out loud and in unison twenty-seven times (they count with a japa mala). After the dance, complete breathing is important to nourish the aura with energy.

8 When they finish, they remain in meditation and begin touching. They touch all over each other's body, especially the neck, mouth, ears, nipples, navel, pubis, sex organs, hands, and legs. This awakens meditative excitement.

9 After a few minutes of caresses, when the kundalini is active and Shakti is ready, she positions herself on top of Shiva in the Yab Yum or Shiva-Shakti pose: she straddles him and is penetrated by Shiva's erect lingam. In this position, with gentle movements in the Way of the Valley, free and deep breathing becomes the thread of energy.

10 The lovers visualize the kundalini like a small reddish-gold thread that unspools from the sacrum up to the head, stimulating the chakras to light up in their corresponding colors.

11 Remember that this is a special ritual and not just another sex act. The slower and deeper the breathing, the less likely it is the man will ejaculate, and both will feel the bioelectric currents circulating through their bodies. The feeling and experience of orgasm will occur several times.

After being mutually satisfied, the lovers stop and begin the final part of the ritual.

"He who practices Tantric Magic needs no drug. The consciousness expands naturally and the Infinite manifests itself."

THE FINAL *RITUAL*

▼ *Visualize a desire, project, material item, spiritual wish, or any other thing you need as a couple. You should see it in your mind's eye, filling the wish with loose energy for several minutes.*

▼ *Lay back, joined sexually in the X pose, and use the secret language (alternating pressure with the PC muscle). With this Yoga Nidra asana you relax the back and sink into peace.*

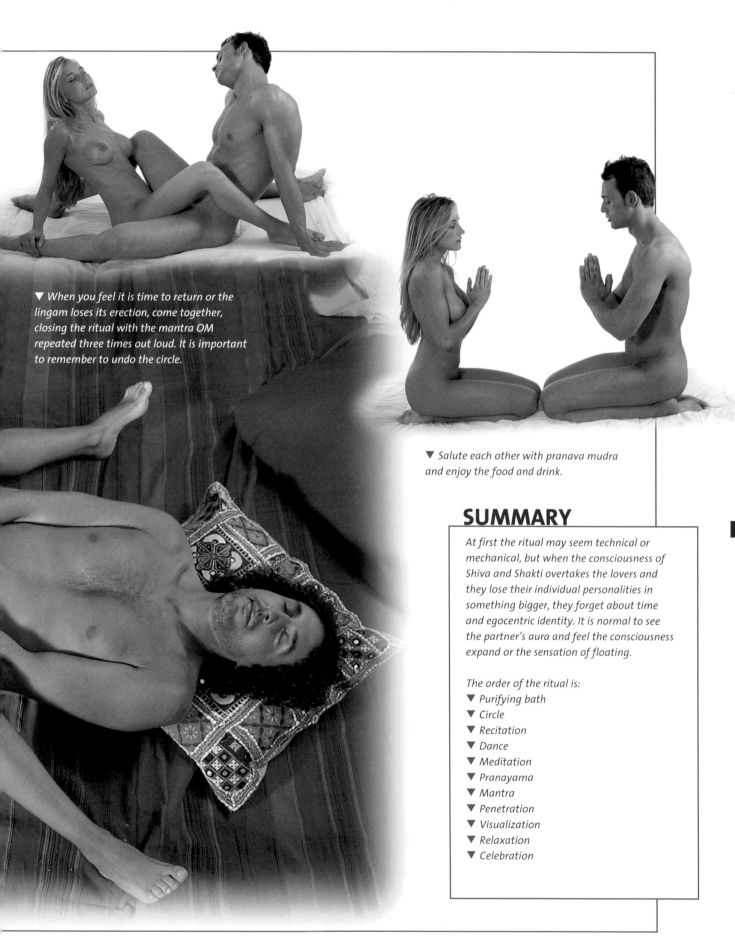

▼ When you feel it is time to return or the lingam loses its erection, come together, closing the ritual with the mantra OM repeated three times out loud. It is important to remember to undo the circle.

▼ Salute each other with pranava mudra and enjoy the food and drink.

SUMMARY

At first the ritual may seem technical or mechanical, but when the consciousness of Shiva and Shakti overtakes the lovers and they lose their individual personalities in something bigger, they forget about time and egocentric identity. It is normal to see the partner's aura and feel the consciousness expand or the sensation of floating.

The order of the ritual is:
▼ Purifying bath
▼ Circle
▼ Recitation
▼ Dance
▼ Meditation
▼ Pranayama
▼ Mantra
▼ Penetration
▼ Visualization
▼ Relaxation
▼ Celebration

Ritual of the *SUN and the* FULL MOON

"If you enchant Shakti, you also enchant the Moon.

If you seduce Shiva, you receive the energy of the Sun."

The three days leading up to the full Moon, the lovers perform the following ritual:

1 Between 9 and 11 at night, they begin to dance naked with music of drums, flutes, and zither, or to flamenco or Arabic music—any melody that incites passion, giving, and sensuality.

2 They dance freely, following the energetic principles of tantric dance: breathing, liberty, and consciousness.

3 After feeling the movement of energy, body heat, and expansion of the aura for at least forty-five minutes, the couple sits face-to-face to begin working on the solar forces, found in the navel (third chakra) and the lunar forces, found in the third eye (sixth chakra).

4 They practice bellow breaths for three minutes and then hold it with jalandhara bandha for fifteen seconds. They release the bandha, breathe completely, and hold it two more times. They consciously swallow the saliva produced, bringing their tongues to their palates.

5 At the same time they begin to visualize the energy in the solar plexus like a tiny Sun that covers the stomach. They should feel the heat melt the lunar fluids in the head and produce "drops of wisdom," a rich energetic substance produced in the pineal and pituitary glands, absorbed through saliva.

6 They visualize a half Moon pointing down, in the area of the third eye, focusing all consciousness and energy in this spot.

7 After completing that step, they begin touching: first, one partner takes the active role and the other relaxes in shavasana. They run their hands from the pubis, over the stomach, chest, throat, and finally the head and forehead, feeling how the energy flows through the body, nourishing it and unblocking the sleeping areas. They should touch in a gentle but sensual manner, letting the sexual energy flood every pore of the partner's skin. If they become excited, they breathe and feel it, but continue the ritual.

8 After a few minutes, they exchange roles.

9 If they have the opportunity, they should look at the moon through a window or do the ritual outside in a natural setting. They must observe the Moon physically before closing their eyes and seeing it with the Third Eye. The full Moon gives the power of psychic and mental openness, and also increases intuition.

For the three days before the full Moon, you should perform this ritual with the objective of accumulating energy and desire, and deepening the consciousness.

Do not perform the sexual act until the day of the full Moon.

OBJECTIVE

Increase internal energy. Awaken inner powers. Absorb the energy of the full Moon. Alchemize the solar and lunar forces.

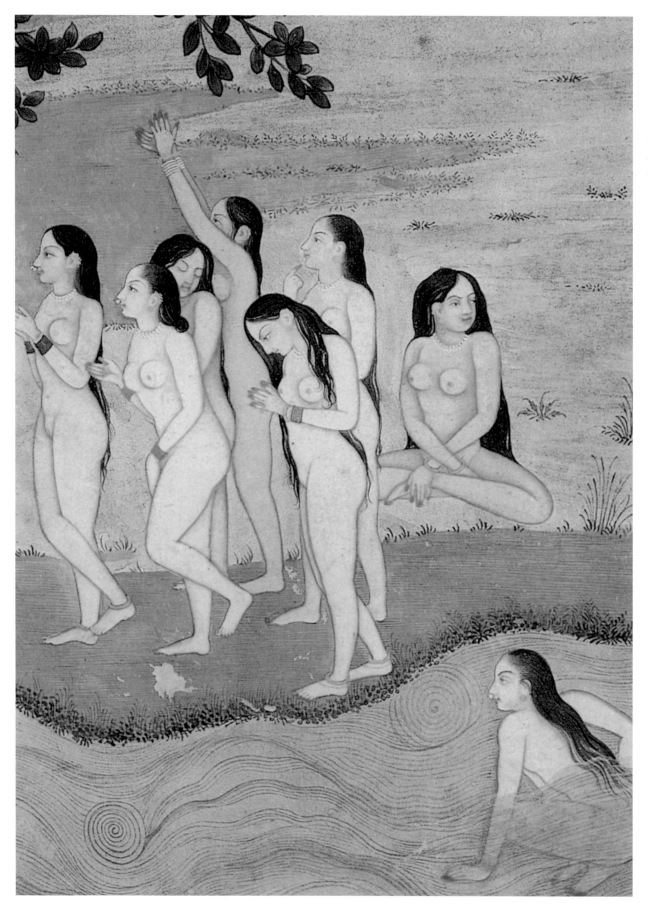

The feminine energy fills ever pore.

NIGHT OF THE FULL MOON

This is the night of Shakti in all her glory. The Moon reflects the light of the Sun in all its splendor, and this combination of forces is absorbed for maximum energy.

▼ The lovers dance naked for twenty minutes, after which they sit and repeat the mantras of the Sun and the Moon for five minutes: RAM, TAM, and OM.

They visualize the solar and lunar forces in the body, the navel, and the Third Eye.

▼ They begin touching the body of the lover gently but with energy. When the kundalini awakens, they let its flow carry them to the peaks of sexual passion, maintaining a meditative state. Remember that the consciousness must be stronger than instinct, so when you feel the enormous wave of energy you must channel it upward through the chakras.

174

The lovers satisfy each other sexually, changing positions, maintaining their preferred rhythm, and breathing the fire produced between the physical and energetic bodies. It is the time to nourish and awaken the chakras through a meditative sexual act. If the animal instinct awakens, you don't have to repress it, just feel it while controlling the rhythm. The man should not ejaculate for any reason during any of these rituals.

▼ After maithuna, for any amount of time (although it is useful to change position every twenty minutes), they lie together "spooning": one lies on their right side and the other behind, embracing them. They repeat the mantra OM a few times out loud but softly, visualizing the solar and lunar forces in the body, and give in to a state of Yoga Nidra until the new day dawns.

▼ The three days following the full Moon, it is useful to meditate in silence, repeat OM, and practice maithuna in the Way of the Valley.

SACRED TEXTS

Goraksashatakam says:

"In the area of the navel there is a burning Sun, while at the base of the palate there is a radiant Moon, full of nectar. The inner Moon looks down and lets its nectar fall; the Sun, with its mouth up, swallows it. In this respect, you should know the secret practices to obtain and conserve this nectar. If a person can preserve the Moon's nectar, their body is no longer affected by physical decline and they remain out of reach of death. What's more, the semen of the yogi whose body is full of this nectar moves upward and gives many miraculous powers."

Shiva Samhita says:

"The sensible yogi should practice khechari mudra to drink the lunar secretions without any loss. Invert the tongue, fix it into the cavity of the throat and carefully position it in the well of nectar that is inside. Know that this is the source of all success. Through this process he controls the micro cosmos and all the things that limit."

Ritual of
PROSPERITY *and*
ABUNDANCE

"All that you sow, you will reap."

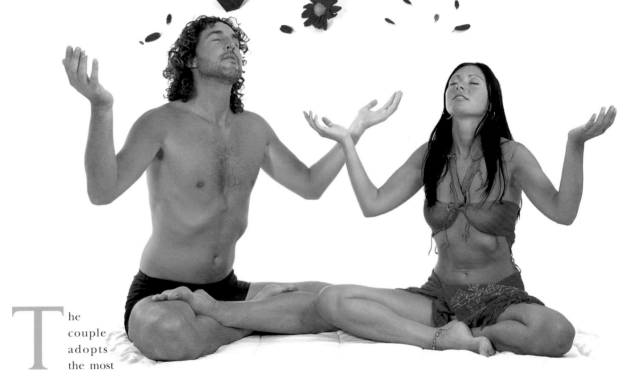

The couple adopts the most comfortable meditation pose, connecting to their center and filling their mind with silence.

Helped by the mantra OM MANI PADME HUM ("God lives within me"), they let the mind subconsciously fill with its meaning. Abundance is a quality of Life and God: there is a variety of landscapes, trees, flowers, fruits, rivers, seas, species . . . Tantra affirms that richness, and the couple visualizes all the marvels of the planet; they go walking through fields of harvest and mentally elaborate what they need, keeping the mental eye focused on it for five minutes. They stop, repeat the mantra nine times, and continue visualized in the wish.

They do this three times during seven days. Following the axiom "the energy follows thought," prosperity and abundance will appear soon.

It is important to know that the ritual is meant to concrete a wish and take in psychomental energy, but afterward you must develop an intelligent plan to work toward its completion. It is also useful to write down the wish and not let any negative emotion or doubt block the power of this ritual.

OBJECTIVE

Assure material well-being.

Ritual of the
KUNDALINI

Kundalini is the motor of life and it sleeps in the first chakra.

When you move your body and your energy, kundalini travels to your soul.

1 The lovers begin laying out the circle and preparing the setting.

2 After doing some Yoga poses to stretch the body and meridians, they do seven complete breaths, seated back-to-back, and ninety bellow breaths in unison. After, they apply the three bandhas: muladhara, uddiyana, and jalandhara, holding their breath three times for fifteen seconds. This increases the temperature in the first chakra.

3 With backs straight, the lovers visualize a small reddish-gold flame in the first chakra that intensifies and progressively unwinds in each chakra. In each chakra they repeat seven times the corresponding mantra; LAM, VAM, RAM, HAM, YAM, and OM, and then "OM NAMAH KUNDALINI" or "OM SHAKTI HUM" for about five minutes.

OBJECTIVE

Awaken the kundalini through maithuna.

4 When it reaches the top of the head, the two remain in silence, feeling their consciousness expand.

5 Using touch, they go over each other's bodies until the psychosexual energy of the kundalini floods the skin, and they practice maithuna in the asanas they prefer, maintaining visualization of energy, breathing, and consciousness at all times. If the couple reaches a point where the man has difficulty controlling ejaculation, they stop, apply the techniques previously taught, and recite the mantra of the kundalini, continuing later.

6 They finish the ritual lowering energy through the forward channel through the third eye, throat, chest, and navel, where it can be stored.

Ritual of the Goddess
KALI

Kali is the sexual initiator, the impassioned one,
she who knows no fear, the terrible, the destroyer, she who transforms
consciousness, she who unveils mysteries.

Kali likes sensual smells like sandalwood, musk, camphor, and patchouli, as well as red flowers, music, dance, and wine. She also likes laughter, songs in her honor, passionate love, and courageous people.

This ritual is done during the dark phase of the Moon:

1 Naked, the lovers salute the four cardinal points—North, South, East, and West—with hands at their chests, while lighting four white candles.

They draw the circle and begin the ritual by reciting the following prayer:

"Kali, naked feminine spirit / necklace of sensual pearls / full of passion and courage. / Kali, you are the initiator of mysteries. / You are the bridge uniting the mundane and the transcendent. / Oh Kali, you are so beautiful and powerful / you are gift of the soul. / You bring Liberation through sex and wisdom.

OBJECTIVE

Connect to Kali's energy and attributes. Destroy the personal ego and reach a higher consciousness through sensuality.

"Kali, Kali, Kali, hold me in your arms goddess / pleasure me in your woman's arms. / You who cuts the head off ego / destroy my weaknesses and strengthen my soul / undress me inside so I can see the Light.

"Your tongue inspires passion and wakens desire / your sword cuts ignorance. / Kali, you feed the kundalini in my body / you are authentic, you grant wishes."

2 In honor of Kali, the lovers offer an erotic and energetic dance that embodies the attributes of the prayer. They seek to connect deeply with their spirit and energy, and visualize how a beautiful woman with long black hair, painted eyes, four arms symbolizing the cardinal points, and a shapely, eternally young body. Her gaze is piercing and powerful, and she is extremely sensual, with her tongue out evoking the fire of sex. Her third eye is open, full of wisdom.

3 They repeat the mantra of Kali ("OM KANG KALIKA NAMAH") for at least half an hour so that her

energy manifests in the woman, although they can also simply repeat the powerful name: "KALI."

4 When the couple thinks they have recited enough, they enter a deeper meditative space, visualizing Kali's yantra, or mystic diagram, which consists of five concentric equilateral triangles, on top of a lotus flower with eight petals. The five triangles of Kali's yantra symbolize the transcendence of the five principle senses and bodily elements. The eight-petal lotus indicates that in order to understand Kali, you must center your emotions in the heart chakra. Therefore, in the center of this yantra you should visualize a small point that is the stability of consciousness; a powerful symbol of meditation and a talisman of protection that you should draw with total devotion and creativity. The wet yoni is also a yantra of Kali, where the pubic hair symbolizes the inverted triangle, her clitoris, the center of consciousness, the sexual odors, the power of enchantment, and secretions, the nature that provides all.

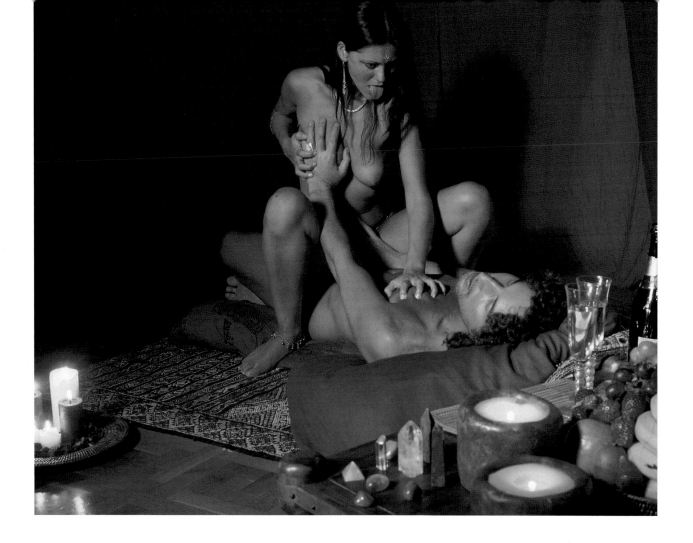

Kali adores the repetition of her mantras and visualization of her yantra, so when she perceives devotion and unity, she gives the ascension of energy and spiritual liberation. Through sexual tantric ritual, the participants can completely transcend karmas and unresolved conflicts in the personality.

5 After visualizing the yantra, the woman holds her feet and lifts her legs until she is balanced on her gluteus. (It's fine if her legs aren't fully outstretched.) Shiva meditates on her naked yoni; he kisses it, honoring the energy it protects (the principle of life), and drinks its highly energetic juices. The goddess doesn't lose her balance, although it's important to have practice with yoga poses to control the body.

6 The man lies face up, relaxing his body, and the woman, fully incarnating Kali, positions herself on top of him. Shiva touches the erotic parts of her body and she touches his; when they feel the desire intensify along with devotion and consciousness of Kali, the woman sticks out her tongue fully, signaling excitement and passion, and inserts the lingam in her wet yoni. They perform maithuna only in this asana, which allows for Kali's undulating movements.

Once the sexual organs unite, they repeat the mantra OM with each exhalation; both when they scale the peaks of passion and ecstasy and when they descend into a subtler connection.

Completely losing individual egos, embodying Shiva and Kali, the couple fulfill themselves sexually and spiritually, until reaching a state of complete silence, bliss, and meditative ecstasy.

7 The lovers close the ritual giving thanks to the energy of the goddess Kali and eating fruits, vegetables, and other light foods, and wine in her honor.

ADVANCED VARIATION

Bhairavi Chakra. This ritual can be done with three, five, seven, or nine participants. One of the women will be the center of the ritual, naked and without intervening and will serve as *the living image of Kali. This woman accepts flowers, fruits, and drink in honor of the goddess, while the other participants complete the mantras, dances, and maithuna.*

Ritual of the Magic Circle: CHAKRA PUJA

This ritual involving more than one couple can create an energetic circle so powerful that it brings a unique experience.

The circle is the symbol of perfection. He who enters the tantric circle unites his inner woman and man, ready to ascend to Absolute Unity.

This sexual ritual is meant to form an extremely powerful energetic circle, in which two or more couples participate ("chakra puja" means "circular worship"). It can also be done solely through visualization but the Left Path of Tantra accepts and practices the whole ritual.

The participants will be guided by a couple that serves as guide and guru.

1 Arranging themselves to sit in a circle, they recite the mantra OM thirty-six times.

OBJECTIVE

Free yourself from taboos and repression. Reach the spiritual dimension of Samadhi. Bring energy to higher vibrations. Create an energetic field to fulfill wishes. Transform consciousness completely. Awaken and empower the chakras with all the abilities they possess.

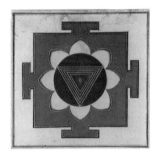

Kali's Yantra

2 Distancing themselves from mundane thoughts, the participants sink into meditation, after which they will start to touch their erogenous zones to awaken the kundalini.

3 One couple begins to make love, and when they reach the climax before orgasm, they stop.

4 Next, another couple does the same, and so on until the wheel has been completed. After this, they all meditate with the enormous energy that has been awakened, and begin the meditative group sex act. This way they create a luminous circle full of vitality and powers, which feeds the psychic centers or chakras of all participants. At all times they practice complete breathing and visualize the chakras, guided by the guru couple, until they reach supraconsciousness in the seventh chakra.

5 The ritual ends with the repetition of the mantra OM thirty-six times.

Tantra teaches that the correct practice of this ritual offers spiritual ecstasy and creative powers, as well as opening access to a new dimension of consciousness.

A VARIATION

For advanced participants: Each woman leaves, at the beginning of the ritual, a personal item (scarf, sock, etc.) and each man chooses one at random to determine who will be his partner in the ritual.

Let it be clear that the focus of Tantra is not a moral one, but it's not an excuse for lack of control or orgy, but rather of courage and wisdom to explore the human being in its totality in search of the transcendent; therefore, the rituals are only successful when the participants do them with sacred consciousness.

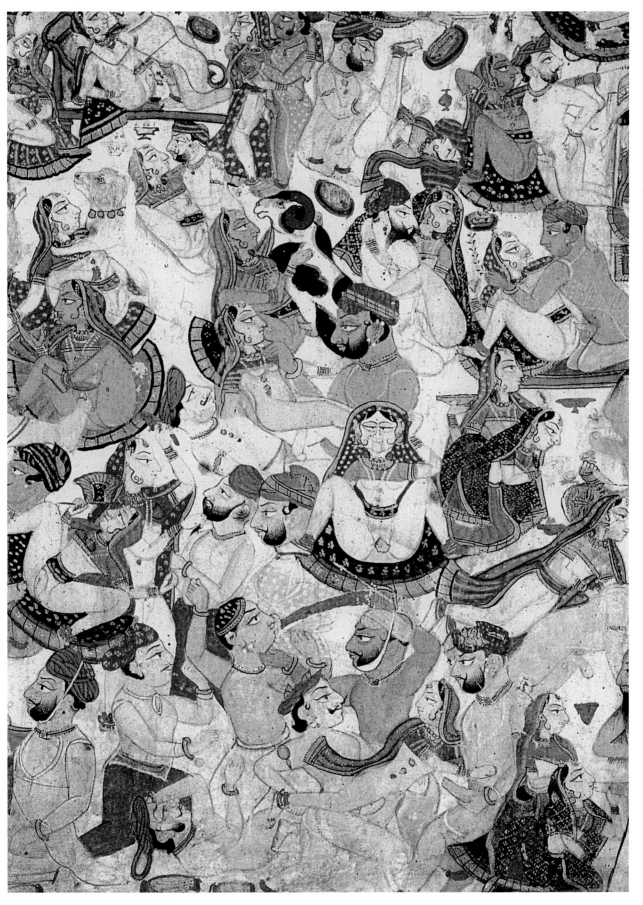

The ritual
involving
various couples
is a magical,
transcendental
encounter that, if
conducted well,
can provide an
experience of
enlightenment
and ecstasy.

Ritual of the MIRROR

"The mirror reveals your original face."

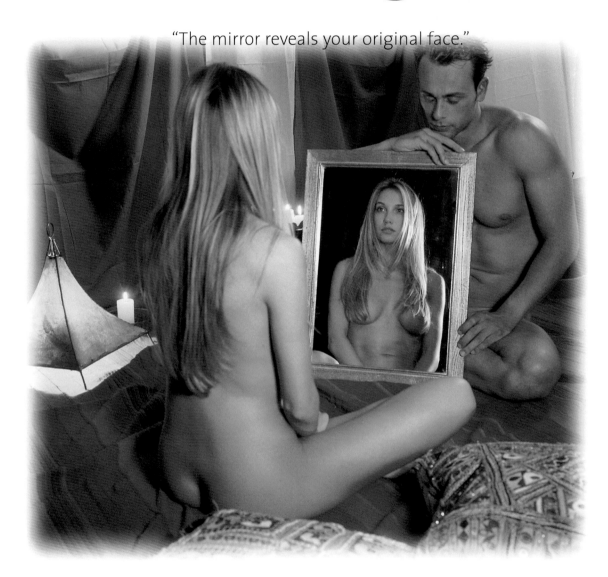

This ritual is done before a new mirror or one that has only reflected your image. Seated in ardha siddhasan (half lotus) with the body naked, the lover

OBJECTIVE

Cease to identify with your physical body. Perceive that beyond our form we are energy.

observes their image in the mirror. Developing impersonal and observational consciousness, they focus their gaze on the eyes until the image fades away. They should practice abdominal or low breathing.

They contemplate their own image and personal energy for a few minutes,

then close their eyes and meditate in silence.

This ritual can be done alone or with your partner. The second option allows two variations: observe the body of the lover as if it were your own, or observe yourselves making love then close your eyes and feel the energy projected in the mirror.

IF THE ENTIRE
WORLD PRACTICED TANTRA

There'd be no lawyers, because there'd be no conflicts.
There'd be no doctors, because there'd be no sickness.
There'd be no insurance salesmen, because there'd be nothing to insure.
There'd be no pharmacies, because we would all be healthy.
There'd be no money, because you'd get everything you wanted.
There'd be no desire, because everything would be yours.
There'd be no sexual taboos, because everyone would live orgasmically.

There'd be no politicians, because there'd be no one to govern.
There'd be no psychologists, because everyone would own their destiny.
There'd be no religions, because God would be laughing in every heart.
There'd be no death, because we'd have powers to see the other planes of life.
There'd be no suffering, because we would be wise.
There'd be no pain, because we'd use our consciousness.
There'd be no notaries, because our word would be enough.

There'd be no bureaucracy, because life would be simple.
There'd be no long faces, because Earth would be a big party.

There'd be no fear, because we would choose to love.
There'd be no states, because we'd realize the Earth belongs to no one.

There'd be no critics, because we would be creating.
There'd be no soap operas or news shows, because we'd experience ecstasy watching the sunset.
There'd be no police, because there'd be no one to control.

There'd be no future preoccupations, because we would enjoy of the present moment.
There'd be no attachments, because we would live traveling.
There'd be no repression, because we would be nude on the beaches.
There'd be no stupid people, because we would all be geniuses.
There'd be no drugs, because we would live in spiritual illumination.
There'd be no clocks, because time would not exist.
There'd be no need to win, because there would not be any competition.
There'd be no need for competition, because we would not have an ego.

And everyone would be a great artist, spiritual and free, creating ideas, books, paintings, music, sculptures, and monuments in eternal honor and thanks to God for the great gift we have received: our own lives.

GUILLERMO FERRARA

FINAL COMMENTS

The method I have created I call "Tantra of the Heart of Fire," since it seeks to "sweep away" everything that blocks you from feeling from the essence—call them fears, doubts, taboos, morals, prejudices, criticism, submission, guilt, beliefs, subconscious, or traumas—so that the human heart recovers playfulness, enthusiasm, vitality, a luminous vision of life, creative projects, celebration, good humor, and consciousness of the internal fire raised above the animal to the human, ready to take the leap into the divine. From there we are conscious that all inner work is focused on stoking that serpentine fire toward the heart to free it.

Regarding the courses and seminars I give about Tantra, many people have been interested and been learning for some years, each time more of them, and in these courses and seminars they practice the techniques and exercises taught here in this book as well as many more they continue to create. Most of them take place on a weekend or a full week, in paradisiacal landscapes surrounded by natural beauty. The benefits of these encounters are numberless, so it is a unique opportunity for self-knowledge and transformation.

Finally, I suggest you remember the sacred character of the subject, but without removing its innocence or burdening it with mysticism, seriousness, or pseudomorality. Sex should stop being connected to morality, since it is an inevitable attraction between opposites: the archetypes of energy beyond the names. It is, definitively, a profound desire to recover lost consciousness, the original One, the loss of ego, the entrance into eternal ecstasy.

QUESTIONS ABOUT MAITHUNA

There are a variety of questions that typically arise about the ritual of maithuna. Since the Tantra I teach is an open door to conscious and meditative sex, in most workshops we don't actually do it, but replace it with the exercise **"the ship of love,"** where you can reach a state of orgasmic ecstasy without compromising the integrity of the participants. In any case, since I work with two modules (for groups of people who don't know each other or personalized lessons for one or more couples who already have experience with energetic spiritual work), **it is possible to practice the ritual**. I'm conscious that maithuna is a sacred act and normally lasts between three and five hours, so the guide, visualizations, specific breathing techniques, and all that goes with it take it well beyond the simple act of "making love." In Tantra, an embrace with secret breathing techniques alone can often deeply affect the sadhakas, so the union of genitals isn't necessary. **Maithuna is a special occasion, magical, sacred, and it can't be properly completed without adequate preparation**, which requires a lot of internal work. **I recommend that couples that have not been together long use condoms and get screened for STIs**, so that there can be greater trust and openness between them. I've taken this as a given, since we are always talking about conscious and intelligent sex.

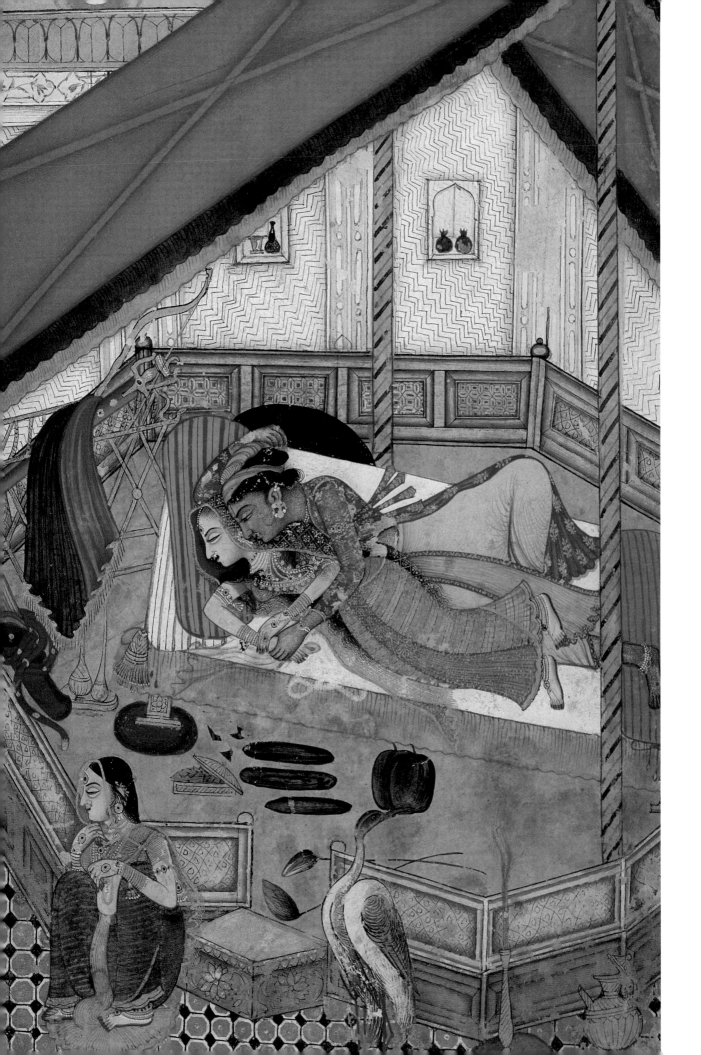

GLOSSARY

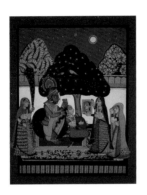

AHAMKARA: individual ego, personality mask

AJNA: sixth chakra, third eye, individual's inner capacity to see clearly

AMRITA: feminine ejaculatory fluid, has energetic properties

ANAHATTA: fourth chakra, linked to emotions and feelings

APANA: energy from the earth

APHRODISIAC: substances that help awaken sexual energy; the most well known are musk, sandalwood, patchouli, cinnamon, oysters, and seafood

AGAMAS: source of teachings related to the rituals, written as a dialogue between Shiva and Parvati

ASANA: psychophysical and spiritual pose

ASVINI MUDRA: dynamic contraction of the anus

ATMA: individual soul

ATMAN: universal soul

ALCHEMY: transformation of magical sexual energy into spiritual power; activity related to the ancient pursuit of turning lead into gold; tantric alchemy is internal, between the components and energetic levels.

ANAHATTA CHAKRA: fourth chakra, meaning "not hit"; the site of loving emotions

ANANDA: bliss, happiness, joy, spiritual ecstasy

ANANDA RANGA: summary of eroticism written in the 16th century by Kalyanamalla

AURA: energetic field around the physical body

BANDHA: energetic lock to elevate the kundalini, produce transformation of energy, and control ejaculation

BHAKTI: devotion

BHOGA: conscious pleasure of the senses, and sensual joy

BIJA: a seed sound, repeated for preparation for meditation

BRAHMA NADI: also call the sushumna andi, the central channel, or cerebrospinal axis; thin as a hair, this is where the kundalini rises from the first chakra up to the brain

BINDU: semen

BRAHAMARANDA: opening in the top of the head where energy enters, and the soul leaves the body in the moment of death

BUDDHA: state of enlightenment of the consciousness; name given to Siddhartha Gautama after enlightenment

CLITORIS: cluster of nerve endings located above the vaginal opening, its purpose only to provide pleasure; in Tantra, it is called "the crown jewel"

CHAKRA: energetic wheel that powers the functions of the psyche

CHAKRA PUJA: circular worship practiced with eight to forty-eight participants guided by an instructor to complete a transcendental magical-energetic ritual

CHAKRASANA: advanced sexual yoga pose to excite energy

CHANDRA: moon

CHANDAMAHAROSANA TANTRA: means "text of the great lunar elixir"

CHITTA: unconscious mind

CHI: name of energy, also prana, ki, or vital essence

DAKINI: feminine demigods that offer the personification of different levels of initiation

DWIJ: spiritual rebirth

DEVA: term to designate a divine being; from this is derived the Western term "diva" to refer to a glamorous woman

DEVA CHAKRA: ritual in which a man celebrates the sexual ritual with five women to stimulate the five senses

DEVI: goddess

DIKSHA: initiation by a spiritual master

DYONISIS: the Greek god of ecstasy, wine, women, sexuality, happiness, and mystic trance; dedicated to expressing his emotions and feelings of fullness and gratitude

DUTI: a dakini that acts as intermediary and sexual initiator

EROS: force of attraction between lovers; one of the types of love, along with Philos, filial love, and Agape, universal love

ESSENCE: name given to the inner center, soul, or divine spark

G-SPOT: area popularized in the West by Dr. Ernest Grafenberg; located in the upper wall of the vagina, it can be felt with a finger; called the "sacred spot" or "point of ecstasy" by tantrics

GANESHA: Hindu god, symbolized with four arms and the head of an elephant; represents spiritual and material success

GOPIS: partners, maidens; name of the 108 lovers of Krishna

GUNAS: the three attributes of material (prakriti) and things; Satva, purity, Rajas, activity, Tamas, inertia

HATHA: sun and moon

IDA: lunar channel

INITIATION: in Tantra there are various types of beginnings in the spiritual path, the sexual ritual is the most important movement of initiation

JALANDHARA BHANDA: lock in the throat to store energy

JAPA: repetition of a seed mantra

KALA CHAKRA: circle of flowers and essences that symbolize the yoni

KALACHAKRA TANTRA: Tantric text from the 7th century describing the phenomena of the world. Also astronomy, geography, and engineering. The secret parts talk about the body, mind, nadis, and sexual meditations.

KALI: the passionate, sensual, and powerful aspect of Shakti; goddess that destroys ego, represents the creative and destructive aspects of nature; embodies desire, liberation, and joy

KALIKA PURANA: tantric text from the 10th century that refers to the worship of the goddess Kali

KALIVILASA TANTRA: text containing information about sexual sadhana

KAMA: desire, delight

KARMA: action (kar) of the mind (man)

KALI YUGA: the age of Kali, the current age

KAMA LOKA: world of desires

KAMA SUTRA: wisdom of desire, ancient Indian text about the secrets of mystic sexuality

KAMAKHYA TANTRA: text describing the power of the yoni

KAULAVALI NIRVAYA TANTRA: text describing sex, social customs, and maithuna

KANDA: energetic oval located below the navel, where all the nadis begin

KUMBHAKA: holding of breath

KUNDALINI: sexual and psychic energy stored in the first chakra, represented by a snake

KHAJURAHO: Indian temples that contain representations of couples in coitus, located in a town of the same name; meant for meditation on the sexual façade so that the mind would be clean before entering inside, where there are no images

KOKA SHASTRA: erotic book from the 12th century, similar to the Kama Sutra (3rd century)

KUBJIKA TANTRA: text about the knowledge of virginity

KULA OR KAULA: left hand school of tantra, or Vamacara

KULARNAVA TANTRA: important work written in the year 1000. Mentions Shakti's questions answered by Shiva

KUMARI TANTRA: work describing sacrifices and the cult of Kali

LAKSHMI: artistic aspect of woman, Brahma's wife

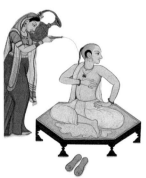

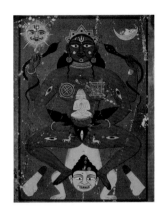

LINGAM: male sexual organ

LILAH: the game of life

LOTUS: sacred flower from India, very beautiful even though it grows in the mud. Yoga pose

MADYA: wine, the ritual drink of maithuna

MAHACINACARA-SARA TANTRA: small text that talks about Buddha and sexual rituals

MAHAMUDRA: the great stamp or symbol; the locking of all the orifices of the body

MAHANIRVANA TANTRA: text translated and introduced to the West by Arthur Avalon

MAITHUNA: mystic sexual ritual to experience spiritual transcendence

MANDALA: geometric diagram that represents a center; a tool for meditation

MANIPURA: third chakra, will power

MANTRA: spiritual sound to quiet and free the mind

MOKSHA: spiritual liberation

MUDRA: hand gesture to channel energy

MULABHANDA: root lock, contraction of the anal sphincter to stimulate the kundalini

MULADHARA: first chakra, home of the kundalini

NADIS: channels where vital energy circulates the energetic body. There are 72,000 of them, fourteen that are most important and well-known due to their relation to organs and physical bodily functions

NIRVANA: extinction of ego, fusion with the consciousness of eternal life

NILA TANTRA: text in which Shiva asks and Parvati answers. Written in the 11th century and refers to rules of purification and the mantras.

NIRUTTARA TANTRA: text that centers exclusively on women and life

NYASA: protection ritual done before maithuna, where you touch certain body parts to seal in energy

OJAS SHAKTI: energy, force, and spiritual power produced by transforming semen and sexual energy

OM: the original sound of the universe

ORGASM: explosion of light in the cells, blissful state where egotistic consciousness disappears to fuse with divinity

ORGY: from Latin "orgia," meaning "state of inspired exaltation," "sacred sexual ceremony"

PADMINI: the lotus woman, prefers to make love during the day

PARVATI: sweet and compassionate aspect of Shakti

PANCHAMAKARA OR PANCHATATTVA: ritual of the five Ms: madya (wine), mamsa (meat), matsya (fish), mudra (gesture), and maithuna (sex)

PARASURAMA-KALPA SUTRA: text of aphorisms about sacred sex

PC MUSCLE: important muscle located in the base of the pelvis, called "pubococcygeus," that in the man helps control ejaculation and in the woman, strengthens the vaginal walls to increase orgasms

PINGALA: solar channel

PRAGNA: intuitive intelligence

PRANA: vital energy

PRAKRITI: term for material

PREMA: love

PRANAYAMAS: techniques for absorbing vital energy

PURAKA: inhalation

RAJAS: active quality of things

RAJA CHAKRA: tantric ritual with one man and five women to power his five senses

RECHAKA: exhalation

SADHAKA: spiritual seeker

SADHANA: spiritual practice, constant exercise

SAHASRARA: seventh chakra, located at the top of the head

SALIVA: important magic element exchanged during sex

SARASVATI: goddess of music, dance, and artistic forms; patron of the sixty-four arts of the kama sutra

SEMEN: chemically irreproducible substance. Sacred bindu is the raw material for the energetic revolution of Tantra. Curiously, the name Jesus or Joshua (Greek and Hebrew) means "semen that heals" or "anointed with semen"

SAMADHI: state of consciousness, of dissolving in the Totality

SAMANA: one of the functions of prana, linked to excretion

SATTVA: luminous and pure quality of things

SECRET LANGUAGE: Tantric communication between the lingam and yoni

SEXUAL MAGIC: tantric teachings about the use of transmuted sexual energy, especially the school of Vamacara

SHAKTI: energy of the feminine principle

SHIVA: energy of the masculine principle

SHIVA SAMHITA: text about yogic study and development. From the 17th century, teaches about anatomy, breathing techniques, and energetic techniques

SHIVA LINGAM: symbolic representation of the penis with stones or other objects

SIDDHIS: extrasensory powers

SURYA: sun

SUSHUMNA: central channel through which the kundalini rises

SUTRAS: aphorisms, teachings

SWADISTHANA: second chakra, linked to sexual energy

TAMAS: heaviness and slowness of things

TANTRA: etymologically, fabric to expand the consciousness. Holistic system of all the functions and activities of the human being, from sexuality to spiritual evolution. Revolutionary system to eliminate repression and taboos. Developed in the East between the 4th and 7th centuries.

TANTRAS: texts containing teachings

TANTRIC DANCE: ritual to awaken energy and modify consciousness

THIRD EYE: the sixth chakra, sees reality clearly; the point where the soul leaves the body in the moment of death

UDANA: one of the functions of prana, linked to digestion

UDDIYANA BANDHA: lock with the elevation of the abdomen, to store energy

VAYU: vital airs

VISHUDDHA: fifth chakra, linked to creativity

VAJRA: "jewel," term referring to the genitals

VIRYA: term for spiritual seed, semen

VAMACARA: the left hand Tantra, which understands real sexual union; followers of this path are called "vamacharis"

VYANA: one of the functions of prana, linked to blood circulation

YAB-YUM: position in which the man sits cross legged and the woman sits on top of him with legs open, embracing. It is an important tantric position for maithuna and meditation in partners.

YIN: feminine essence

YANG: masculine essence

YOGI: male practitioner of yoga

YOGINI: female practitioner of yoga

YOGINI TANTRA: text about the worship of the goddesses Kali and Kamakhya. Unknown author and date

YANTRA: technique of visualizing powerful objects

YOGA: various energetic paths to integrate the individual consciousness with the Cosmos

YONI: female sexual organ

YONI PUJA: worship of the sacred portal of life, the vagina

YONI TANTRA: text dedicated to creating and consuming the yoni fluids

RECOMMENDED READING

• *TANTRA: THE CULT OF THE FEMININE*
Andre Van Lysebeth

• *SEXUAL SECRETS: THE ALCHEMY OF ECSTASY*
Nik Douglas
and Penny Slinger

• *TANTRA, SPIRITUALITY, AND SEX*
Osho

• *TANTRIC QUEST: AN ENCOUNTER WITH ABSOLUTE LOVE*
Daniel Odier

189

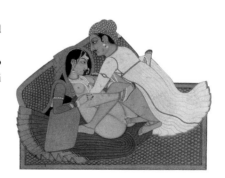

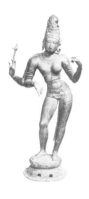 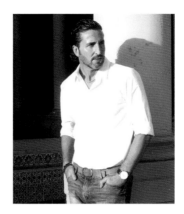

ABOUT THE AUTHOR

Guillermo Ferrara is an artist, therapist, and philosopher, as well as the author of twenty-two books, including several bestselling novels and works on personal development. His books have been translated into Spanish, English, Greek, French, Chinese, German, Portuguese, Serbian, Russian, and Romanian. His books are valuable tools for people to improve their quality of life. A researcher of ancient civilizations and cultures, Ferrara also specializes in holistic philosophy and transpersonal psychology. He teaches about spirituality, tantra, quantum physics, meditation, yoga, alchemical sexuality, emotional healing, and advances in the field of consciousness, from a spiritual-scientific angle.

Ferrara has been an instructor of tantric yoga since 1991. Thousands of people have taken his personal transformation workshops, both in person and online. He has taught courses and conferences in Mexico, the United States, Spain, Greece, London, Germany, Argentina, Colombia, Costa Rica, and several countries where he is contracted to share his extensive experience and his revolutionary method of spiritual enlightenment. He writes articles for newspapers and is frequently invited to present on television and radio.

He is the author of these books, also from Skyhorse Publishing: The New Art of Massage (Skyhorse, 2015), The Ultimate Guide to Tantric Sex (Skyhorse, 2016), and Yoga for Couples (Skyhorse, 2016). He lives in Miami Beach with his wife Sandra.

You may connect with Guillermo Ferrara at:

tantra09@hotmail.com
www.guillermoferrara.org
www.facebook.com/guillermoferrarainUSA
www.twitter.com/GuilleFerrara